E. Jacquelyn Kirkis, R.N., B.S.N., M.Sc., C.I.C.

Seminar Consultant, ECHOES Seminars in Infection Control and Epidemiology
Santa Ana, California
Membership Chair, Association for Practitioners in Infection Control
Orange, California
Director-At-Large, California League for Nursing, N.L.N.

Marya Grier, R.N., B.S.N., M.S.

Nurse Epidemiologist, St. Joseph's Hospital
Independent Infection Control Consultant
Past President, Association for Practitioners in Infection Control
Orange, California

Nurse's Guide to
INFECTION CONTROL PRACTICE

1988
W. B. SAUNDERS COMPANY
Harcourt Brace Jovanovich, Inc.

Philadelphia   London   Toronto   Montreal   Sydney   Tokyo

W. B. SAUNDERS COMPANY
Harcourt Brace Jovanovich, Inc.

West Washington Square
Philadelphia, PA 19105

Library of Congress Cataloging-in-Publication Data

Kirkis, E. Jacquelyn.

Nurse's guide to infection control practice.

Bibliography: p.

1. Communicable diseases—Nursing.   2. Asepsis
and antisepsis. I. Grier, Marya.   II. Title.
[DNLM: 1. Communicable Disease Control—nurses'
instruction.   2. Cross Infection—prevention &
control—nurses' instruction.   WX 167 K59n]

RT95.K57   1988   610.73'699   87-26436

ISBN 0-7216-2373-5

Cover art modified from a design by David Gomez.

Editor: Michael Brown
Designer: Patti Maddaloni
Production Manager: Peter Faber
Manuscript Editor: Kate Mason
Page Layout Artist: Patti Maddaloni

Nurse's Guide to Infection Control Practice

ISBN 0-7216-2373-5

Last digit is the print number: 9   8   7   6   5   4   3   2   1

This reference book is dedicated
to the fiber of perseverance that ensures success at any age
and in the face of any adversity.

PREFACE

The *Nurse's Guide to Infection Control Practice* emphasizes the cost-effective approach, using nursing diagnosis in guides for daily care of infected patients. The guides can be used in any setting for patient care.

E. Jacquelyn Kirkis, RN
Marya Grier, RN

CONTENTS

Nurse's Guide to
INFECTION CONTROL PRACTICE

INTRODUCTION

Infection control in day-to-day patient care is the responsibility of the professional nurse. This is not a written directive but rather a tradition of nursing practice. Early nursing developed, implemented, and taught barrier techniques for the prevention of the spread of disease and infections. Over time, these techniques evolved into "traditions." However, the reasons for their effectiveness were lost because of nursing's inability to relate these procedures to scientific data, and these originally simple, effective barriers became complicated. Nursing, because of a lack of understanding of the transmission of communicable diseases, developed extraordinary methods for taking care of patients with these diseases. In fact, until recently, nursing research into the cause of infectious disease or its transmission has been practically non-existent. Most of our understanding of infectious disease has come from scientific investigation and research done by physicians and medical microbiologists, which have yielded a wealth of information regarding the agents that cause disease: the epidemiology and methods of disease transmission.

A review of current nursing literature shows that many nursing texts are still lacking information on infection control based on scientific research. Therefore, this reference has been designed to assist the nurse to use the available scientific information on infection control in day-to-day patient care. The purpose of the text is to reinforce effective barrier nursing, which is the basis of infection control, with updated research on cost-effective prevention of disease and infection transmission. The information is presented using an alphabetical arrangement of body systems: circulatory, gastrointestinal, genitourinary, integumentary, musculoskeletal, neurological, and respiratory. The diseases seen in these systems are also listed alphabetically. Information regarding immunocompromised patient care and a section concerning miscellaneous infections are also included. The procedures or required conditions for control of each disease or infection are described in a simple chart designed for the infected body system.

The infection control guidelines in this text were developed using Centers for Disease Control (CDC) recommendations and other recognized research in infection control. The CDC has recently published two alternatives for a choice in use of supplies, space, and environment. These choices are (1) category specific and (2) disease specific precautions. This reference can be used with either category. Descriptions of these two categories follow. The format of the charts in this reference allows the nurse and other health care practitioners flexibility in choosing the infection control measures (i.e., category specific or disease specific) that are appropriate for the patient within the policies of the institution.

Each section addresses the important concern of cost effectiveness. Each section uses an "HAA" approach: Handwashing, Assessment, Action. This approach appears in the nursing system analysis as recognition of cause of infection, results of care program, and guides for action.

Disease specific isolation considers each infectious disease individually so that only equipment that is absolutely necessary to interrupt the transmission or the disease is used. Patient care personnel must utilize more skill and responsibility when assigning precautions and must have more diagnostic information about the disease. This form of infection control encourages greater compliance because it minimizes unnecessary precautions and may, therefore, be more cost effective. A single card, individualized for each patient, is used.

Category specific isolation groups diseases into categories. Each category (described below) includes diseases that require similar infection control measures. There is a color-coded card for each category. This system is simple to use because less information and less decision making is needed to assign the necessary precautions. It is a more costly form of infection control because unnecessary precautions may be taken for some diseases placed in a general category.

Strict isolation (SI) prevents transmission of highly contagious or virulent infections that are spread by both air and contact.

1. Private room; door closed.
2. Masks, gowns, gloves.
3. Discard contaminated disposable articles; bag and send reuseables for reprocessing.
4. Good handwashing technique before and after patient care and after handling contaminated articles.

Contact isolation (CI) prevents transmission of highly transmissible or epidemiologically important infections that are spread primarily by direct contact.

1. Private room; patients infected with the same organism may share a room.
2. Masks worn when close to patient.
3. Gowns if soiling likely.
4. Gloves if touching infective material.
5. Discard contaminated disposable articles; bag and send reuseables for reprocessing.
6. Good handwashing technique before and after patient care and after handling contaminated articles.

Respiratory isolation (RI) prevents transmission of infectious diseases over short distances through the air (droplet transmission) by direct or indirect contact.

1. Private room; patients with same organism may share room.
2. Masks worn when close to patient.
3. NO gowns or gloves.
4. Discard contaminated disposable articles; bag and send reuseables for reprocessing.
5. Good handwashing technique before and after patient care and after handling contaminated articles.

Tuberculosis (AFB) isolation prevents transmission of pulmonary and laryngeal TB in patients with positive sputum smear or suggestive chest x-ray.

1. Private room with special ventilation, keep door closed; patients infected with active tuberculosis may share room.
2. Masks if patient is coughing and doesn't cover mouth well.
3. Gowns only if gross contamination is likely.
4. NO gloves.

5. Discard contaminated disposable articles; bag and send reuseables for reprocessing.
6. Good handwashing technique before and after patient care and after handling contaminated articles.

Enteric precautions (EP) prevent infections transmitted by direct or indirect contact with feces.

1. Private room if patient hygiene poor.
2. NO masks.
3. Gowns if soiling is likely.
4. Gloves if touching infective material.
5. Discard contaminated disposable articles; bag and send reuseables for reprocessing.
6. Good handwashing technique before and after patient care and after handling contaminated articles.

Drainage/secretion precautions (D/S) prevent infections transmitted by direct or indirect contact with purulent material or with drainage from an infected body site.

1. NO private room.
2. NO masks.
3. Gowns if soiling is likely.
4. Gloves if touching infected material.
5. Discard contaminated disposable articles; bag and send reuseables for reprocessing.
6. Good handwashing technique before and after patient care and after handling contaminated articles.

Blood/body fluid precautions (B/BF) prevent infection transmitted by direct or indirect contact with infective blood or body fluids.

1. Private room if hygiene is poor or environmental contamination with blood is likely.
2. NO masks, unless aerosolization, i.e., suctioning, or splashing is likely.
3. Gowns if soiling is likely.
4. Gloves if touching blood or body fluids.
5. Discard contaminated disposable articles; bag and send reuseables for reprocessing.
6. Good handwashing technique before and after patient care and after handling contaminated articles.
7. Avoid needle-stick injuries. Handle needles and sharps carefully.
8. Clean up blood spills promptly with 5.25% sodium hypochlorite (bleach) diluted 1:10 with water.

Handwashing is the most cost-effective, practice-effective method to reduce the spread of infection. A current CDC recommendation states that for most activities a vigorous, brief (at least 10 seconds) rubbing together of all surfaces of lathered hands, followed by rinsing under a stream of water, is adequate. The key to good handwashing is thorough, vigorous rubbing. Note: Gloves may be used if there is contact with any blood or body fluid.

Assessment is the assessing of each body system for signs and symptoms of infection (purulent drainage, redness, swelling, heat, and pain) and determining if positive laboratory culture reports are indicative of actual infection or merely colonization. When patients are colonized, they must continue to be observed, since this may lead to infection. If the disease is extensive or the patient is compromised by treatments or procedures, colonization can easily become infection. Assessment includes identification of the infective material as well as of the mode of transmission.

Action/Outcome uses proven cost-effective procedures to prepare the patient, the environment, and supplies to control the transmission of infective agents to other patients and to personnel.

Terms Used In Charts

AF   Acid fast. Organisms that are not easily decolorized by acid after staining.

Bacteremia   Bacteria in the blood shown by positive blood cultures.

Colonization   Presence of organisms on or in the body without invasion or tissue damage. Colonization can lead to infection if the patient is placed at risk through procedures or injury.

Community-acquired infections   Infections incubating at the time of admission to the hospital. They serve as a potential source of infection to other patients and personnel.

Disinfection   Process of destruction of all microorganisms except spores by exposure to a chemical agent, usually a liquid.

ECF   Extended care facility.

Endogenous   Produced or arising from within. Endogenous infections are caused by the patient's own flora.

Exogenous Originating outside an organ or part. Exogenous infections result from the transmission of organisms from a source other than the patient.

Gram-negative (GN) Refers to organisms that take up a red stain.

Gram-positive (GP) Refers to organisms that take up a purple stain.

HIV (Human immunodeficiency virus) Virus that attacks the immune system, making it non-functional; the infected individual has no resistance to opportunistic infections. There is no cure for the infection; there is no treatment to reactivate the immune system. Formerly called HTLVIII/LAV virus (named for the human T-lymphotrophic virus type III).

Immunosuppressed host Patient who is unable to produce an immune system response to an invading organism. Because they lack the signs and symptoms of infection, such patients present a more difficult picture of assessment. This decreased response may be caused by treatment modalities or by disease.

Infection Invasion by a pathogenic agent (microorganism or virus) that, under favorable conditions, multiplies and produces effects that are injurious to tissue.

Microorganisms Bacteria, fungi, viruses, parasites, rickettsia.

Multiply resistant organisms Organisms that are resistant to two or more unrelated antibiotics to which they are normally considered susceptible. Organisms can become multiply resistant through misuse or abuse of antibiotics. (Laboratory culture results are a key factor in conscientious antibiotic therapy.)

Normal flora Microorganisms normally found in a system. Some systems are sterile.

Nosocomial infection Infections that develop within the hospital or are caused by organisms acquired in the hospital.

No touch technique Handwashing prior to dressing change and no contact with wound or wound drainage except with sterile dressings.

Pathogen Microorganism capable of producing infection. All bacteria have the potential to be pathogenic.

Pus Liquid product of inflammation consisting of white blood cells. Pus is a major indication of the presence of infection.

Septicemia Bacteremia associated with the clinical signs and symptoms including chills, fever, petechiae, pustules, and abscesses.

SNF Skilled nursing facility.

Sterile Free from living microorganisms including spores.

Sterilization Process of destruction of all microorganisms including spores by exposure to chemical agents.

Susceptibles Persons who have not had the infection or who are immunosuppressed.

Bibliography

Altmeier, WA; Burke, JF; Pruitt, BA; Sandusky, WR: *Manual on Control of Infection in the Surgical Patient*, 2nd ed. J. B. Lippincott, Philadelphia, 1984.

American Academy of Pediatrics. Committee on fetus and newborn. Committee on infectious diseases. Perinatal herpes simplex virus infections. *Pediatrics* 66:147-149, 1980.

Beaty, HM, MD: *The Central Nervous System; Meningitis Hospital Infections*. Little, Brown & Co., Boston, 1979.

Brunner, LS; Suddarth, DS. (eds.): *Lippincott Manual of Nursing Practice*. J. B. Lippincott, Philadelphia, 1980.

Boyer, AS, MD: Osteomyelitis. In Yoshikawa, T. et al. (eds.). *Infectious Diseases and Management*. Houghton Mifflin, Boston, 1980.

C D C Guidelines for prevention of nosocomial infections. *Am. J. Infect. Control*, 4:4, 1983.

California State Department of Health Services: *Control of Communicable Diseases in California*. American Health Assoc., 1983.

Cruckshank, D, et al. (eds.): *Medical Microbiology*, vols. 1 and 2. Churchill Livingstone, Inc. New York, 1979, 1984.

Franco, JA, MD; Enneking, WF, MD: Infections of skeletal prostheses. In Bennet, JV; Brachman, PS (eds.). *Hospital Infections*. Little, Brown & Co., Boston, 1979.

Haley, W; *Managing Hospital Infection Control for Cost-Effectiveness*. American Hospital Publishing, Inc.., 1986.

Jackson, MM, RN; Lynch, P, RN: Isolation practices: A historical perspective. *Am. J. Infect. Control*, 13:21–31, 1985.

Kilbrick, S: Herpes simplex infection at term. *JAMA*, 243:157-60, 1980.

Paterson, PY, MD: Infection in the compromised host, In Youmans, G.P. et al., (eds.). *The Biologic and Clinical Basis of Infectious Disease*. W. B. Saunders, Philadelphia, 1980.

Robinson, GV, RN, MSPH: Assessment and Criteria of Infection in the Neutropenic Patient. APIC Educational Conference, Orange County, California, June 6, 1984.

Robinson, GV, et al.: Nosocomial Infection in a Cancer Center. APIC Educational Conference, Orange County, California, June 6, 1984.

Sattar, F, MD: *Concise Handbook of Respiratory Diseases*. Reston, Inc., Reston, Virginia, 1978.

Soule, BM, RN, MSN (ed.): *APIC Curriculum For Infection Control Practice*, vol. 1, Kendall/Hunt, Dubuque, Iowa, 1983.

Stark, JL, RN; Hunt, V, RN: Don't let nosocomial infections get your patients down. *Nursing 85*, January 1985.

CIRCULATORY SYSTEM
Guide to Control Infections

Includes Human Immunodeficiency Virus (HIV) (AIDS) Controls

The circulatory system consists of the heart and blood vessel network in the body. The lymphatic system occupies less distinct channels; the lymph flows through nodal junctions and is the same fluid that bathes the tissues. The lymph and tissue fluids are secondary fluids making up the circulatory system. This system has no normal flora. All three fluids (blood, lymph, and tissue fluids) are sterile.

Trauma, surgery, disease, or infection, at any location in the body may spread pathogenic organisms into the blood, the lymph, or the tissue fluid. Placement of prosthetic heart valves, or joints, and transplants are high-risk procedures that can lead to contamination of the circulatory system. Contamination of this system is a potential hazard of infection for other body systems.

Therapeutic manipulations (e.g., surgery) that traumatize mucous membranes or create wounds and the use of intravascular devices (e.g., intravenous (IV) catheters) also contribute to infections of this system.

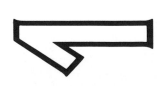

Trauma is particularly dangerous. When deep contusions occur, microorganisms are released from normal locations, such as the gut, into the circulatory system. This can cause sepsis, localized node edema, pain, and pockets of purulence. Deep contusions where the skin is unbroken can be the foci for anaerobic infections such as gangrene.

IN CIRCULATORY INFECTIONS, THE INFECTIOUS MATERIAL IS BLOOD, LYMPH, OR TISSUE FLUID.

HANDWASHING IS ESSENTIAL:
- *Before and after the care of each patient.*
- *If hands come in contact with blood or body fluids.*
- *Before and after performing venipuncture.*
- *Before and after all dressing changes.*

Circulatory System

SITE	ORGANISMS	TYPE STAIN	RELATED DISEASES	SIGNS AND SYMPTOMS
Heart and blood vessels	No normal flora			
	Any microorganism— bacteria, viruses, fungi, parasites—can be a pathogen; normal skin flora can cause bacteremia and sepsis	as nec. for ID	Bacteremia	Bacteremia, as by blood cultures
			Sepsis	Elevated WBC count
				Fever, chills, hypothermia
				Swollen lymph nodes
				Arthralgia
				Cellulitis
				Oliguria
				Hypotension
				Disorientation
				Skin rash

NOTES

SAMPLE AND INSTRUCTIONS FOR
CHARTS FOR HOSPITAL, HOME, OFFICE, AND OUTPATIENT CLINIC

Charts for Hospital, Home, Office, and Outpatient Clinic

DISEASE SPECIFIC CODES

ALL	At all times	SL	If soiling likely
D	Desirable, but optional	SUS	If susceptible
PH	Poor hygiene	WC	With contact

DISEASE	CATEGORY SPECIFIC		DISEASE SPECIFIC						
	Type	Duration	Handwashing—Thorough rubbing, Lather, rinsing	Private Room Needed	Masks	Gowns	Gloves	Linen—if soiled, separate	Containers for Body Fluids; precautions if Contaminated
Common cold									
Adults	-	-	ALL	-	-	-	-	-	-
Infants and children	CI	DI	ALL	ALL	-	SL	-	-	-

HOW TO READ THIS CHART

Steps	Example
1. Locate infection or disease; read from left to right.	Read first row across as: **Common cold in adults** requires *no* special precautions or supplies; *handwashing* is required to prevent transmission.
2. **Type** indicates *Category Specific* control measures.	
3. **Duration** signifies length of time to use *Category Specific* control measures.	
4. Use legend in upper left-hand corner to interpret codes in *Disease Specific* columns.	Read second row across as: **Common cold in infants and children** can require *contact isolation* for duration of infection; *handwashing* is required to prevent transmission; *private room and gloves* are recommended.
5. Column headings in the *Disease Specific* section indicate procedures, patient area, and supplies to be used with *Disease Specific* control measures.	

CATEGORY SPECIFIC CODES

	Type		Duration
AFB	Tuberculosis (AFB) isolation	**CN**	Off antibiotics; culture negative
		DH	Duration of hospitalization
B/BF	Blood/body fluid precautions	**DI**	Duration of illness/drainage
		U-a	Until 24 hours after therapy begins
CI	Contact isolation	**U-b**	Until 2 weeks after therapy begins or until sputa negative
D/S	Drainage/secretion precautions	**U-c**	For 9 days after swelling
		U-d	For 7 days after rash or swelling or onset of infection
EP	Enteric precautions	**U-e**	For 3 days after therapy begins
RI	Respiratory precautions	**U-f**	For 4 days after rash begins; if immunosuppressed, use DI
SI	Strict isolation	**U-g**	Until HBsAg (hepatitis B surface antigen) is negative
		U-h	For 48 hours after effective therapy begins

Charts for Hospital, Home, Office, and Outpatient Clinic

DISEASE SPECIFIC CODES

ALL At all times	**SL** If soiling likely	
D Desirable, but optional	**SUS** If susceptible	
PH Poor hygiene	**WC** With contact	

DISEASE	CATEGORY SPECIFIC				DISEASE SPECIFIC				
	Type	Duration	Handwashing—Thorough Rubbing, Lather, Rinsing	Private Room Needed	Masks	Gowns	Gloves	Linen—if Soiled, separate	Containers for Body Fluids; Precautions if Contaminated
Acquired immunodeficiency syndrome (AIDS)[1,2]	B/BF	DI	ALL	PH	–	SL	WC	ALL	ALL
Arthropod-borne fevers (dengue, yellow fever, Colorado tick fever)	B/BF	DH	ALL	–	–	–	WC	ALL	ALL
Babesiosis	B/BF	DI	ALL	–	–	–	WC	ALL	ALL
Colorado tick fever	B/BF	DH	ALL	–	–	–	WC	ALL	ALL
Creutzfeldt-Jakob disease[1]	B/BF	DH	ALL	–	–	–	WC	ALL	ALL
Dengue fever	B/BF	DH	ALL	–	–	–	WC	ALL	ALL
Hemorrhagic fevers (e.g., Lassa fever)[3]	SI	DI	ALL	ALL	ALL	ALL	ALL	ALL	ALL
Hepatitis—viral									

Type B (serum hepatitis)—includes HB antigen carrier (HBAg+)	B/BF	U-g	ALL	–	–	SL	WC	ALL	ALL
Type non A-non B or unspecified	B/BF	DI	ALL	–	–	SL	WC	ALL	ALL
Unspecified, consistent with viral etiology[4]	–	–	ALL	–	–	–	–	–	–
Jakob-Creutzfeldt disease[1]	B/BF	DH	ALL	–	–	–	WC	ALL	D
Lassa fever[3]	SI	DI	ALL	ALL	ALL	ALL	ALL	ALL	ALL
Leptospirosis[5]	B/BF	DH	ALL	–	–	–	WC	ALL	ALL
Malaria	B/BF	DI	ALL	–	–	–	WC	ALL	D
Marburg Virus Disease[5]	SI	DI	ALL	ALL	ALL	ALL	ALL	ALL	ALL
Rat-bite fever									
Streptobacillus moniliformis	B/BF	U-a	ALL	–	–	–	WC	ALL	ALL
Spirillum minus	B/BF	U-a	ALL	–	–	–	WC	ALL	ALL
Relapsing fever	B/BF	DI	ALL	–	–	–	WC	ALL	ALL
Syphilis[7]	B/BF	U-a	ALL	–	–	–	WC	ALL	D
	& D/S		ALL	–	–	–	WC	ALL	ALL

1. Use caution handling blood and blood-soiled articles, brain tissue, or spinal fluid. For GI bleeding use gloves. Avoid needle sticks: See MMWR, 34:681–686, 691–695, 1985.
2. See Cost-Effective Measures for HIV (AIDS)-Infected Patient, this chapter.
3. Call State Health Department and Centers for Disease Control for advice about management.
4. Maintain precautions for most likely infection.
5. Urine is infective.
6. Respiratory secretions are infective.
7. Skin lesions of secondary and tertiary syphilis may be highly infective.

Sample Nursing Care Guide

RECOGNITION OF CAUSE OF INFECTION	RESULTS OF CARE PROGRAM	GUIDES FOR ACTION
1. Transmission of infectious material: Blood or body fluids.	1. Patient will not become septic.	1. Vital signs will be monitored p.r.n.
2. Laboratory report of positive culture for disease process.	2. IV site will not become infected.	2. Venipuncture will be done aseptically and according to facility policy. Check site daily. Change peripheral cannulas every 48 to 72 hours provided no IV-related complications requiring cannula removal are encountered before this. Sites may be used longer if no other site can be found. Change tubings routinely according to facility policy.
3. Signs and symptoms. ☐ fever ☐ chills ☐ hypotension ☐ hypothermia ☐ oliguria ☐ aberration of mental function ☐ respiratory alkalosis	3. Surgical wound will heal without infection.	3. Change all surgical dressings using NO TOUCH TECHNIQUE p.r.n.
	4. Any abnormal reaction will be evaluated for sepsis.	4. Nursing will correlate the various support systems needed to provide counseling for patient and family, including social services, psychiatry, chaplain, and others as needed.
	5. Counseling will be available to provide support regarding life-style risks for infection or limitations if dyscrasias are identified.	
4. Knowledge deficit of patient or care givers in home or hospital regarding method of infection transmission.	6. Current cost-effective infection control measures will be demonstrated daily in patient care practices.	
	7. Infectious material and equipment will be handled and disposed of properly to prevent transmission.	

Sample Discharge Guide

GENERAL POINTS FOR DISCHARGE	GUIDE FOR CARE IN A CLINIC OR NON-HOSPITAL SETTING	GUIDE FOR CARE IN HOME	GUIDE FOR CARE IN SNF
Information to transmit to anyone receiving a patient with a circulatory infection:	1. Use thorough handwashing before and after all patient care.	1. Use thorough handwashing before and after taking care of patient.	1. Use thorough handwashing before and after all patient care.
1. Identify the source of infection: blood and body fluids.	2. Use gloves if there is a possibility of CONTACT with blood or body fluids.	2. Use gloves if contact with infectious material is possible. *Note:* Gloves are an expensive item for use in the home by family members. Handwashing if done conscientiously has proved to be sufficient in the home.	2. Use gloves if there is a possibility of CONTACT with blood or body fluids.
2. Describe the method of transmission and the infection control measures necessary to prevent contact with infectious material.	3. Use gowns if there is extensive drainage or soiling of clothing is likely.		3. Use gowns if soiling is likely.
	4. Handle dressings carefully. Use NO TOUCH TECHNIQUE.	3. No special precautions are necessary for linens or dishes.	4. No special precautions necessary for linen or dishes.
3. Review all medications prescribed.	5. Dispose of needles and syringes carefully. Do not recap or clip needles.	4. Handle dressings carefully. Use NO TOUCH TECHNIQUE when changing dressings.	5. Handle dressings carefully. Use NO TOUCH TECHNIQUE.
4. Notify any agency or transport personnel of special precautions needed to prevent contact with infectious material.	6. Place soiled dressings in plastic or heavy paper bag. Tie or seal and place in trash.	5. Place soiled dressings in plastic or heavy paper bag, tie or seal, and dispose of in trash.	6. Place soiled dressings in plastic or heavy paper bag, tie or seal and dispose of in trash.
	7. Use regular toilet for disposal of liquid or solid body waste.	6. Use regular toilet for disposal of liquid or solid body waste.	7. Use regular toilet for disposal of liquid or solid waste.
5. Inform public health department if the infection is reportable.	8. If spills or soiling occur, clean surfaces promptly. Use bleach solution diluted 1:10 with water.	7. Use apron or clean towel if soiling of clothing is likely.	8. Dispose of needles and syringes carefully. Do not recap or clip needles.
		8. Clean surfaces with bleach solution diluted 1:10 with water.	9. If spills or soiling occur, clean surfaces promptly. Use bleach solution diluted 1:10 with water.

1

Cost-Effective Measures

The use of proven infection control measures, not rituals, to care for patients with communicable diseases is cost effective. When nursing consistently applies these measures in the health care setting, they reduce infections and death, reduce costs for the facility and patient, reduce potential for malpractice suits, facilitate the accreditation process, and strengthen the infection control program as a whole.

When the patient is hospitalized, the following guidelines must be used:

1. Use good handwashing technique at all times.
2. IV therapy should be used only when therapeutically or diagnostically indicated.
3. Wash hands before and after any manipulation of catheter site or apparatus.
4. Use careful insertion technique:
   - Avoid cutdowns.
   - Use the upper extremities rather than lower.
   - Prepare skin properly, per established procedure; DO NOT USE aqueous benzalkonium-like compounds or hexachlorophene.
   - Always use aseptic technique.
5. IV site should be inspected every 24 hours.
6. Remove cannula if there are signs of infection; obtain a gram stain and culture of any pus. Culture the catheter, tubing, and fluid.
7. Change cannulas every 48 to 72 hours; change IV administration set per current protocol. Heparin lock may remain in site as long as patent and trouble-free.

8. Maintain the sterile integrity of the system, including the fluid, stopcocks, and transducers.

9. Reduce use of stopcocks in intravenous system.

When the patient is cared for at home, optimum clean techniques are acceptable. The simplest methods to keep the home clean, orderly, and safe are the most practical and cost-effective methods. Rarely will it be necessary to take the "sterile" emphasis into the home. The patient will be returning to a known environment where there will be few if any unusual organisms. Handwashing and NO TOUCH TECHNIQUE are the most important factors to emphasize in the home for wound care and drainage secretion and excretion control. These optimum clean techniques will prevent transmission of infective material.

Sample Nursing Care Guide for the Patient with Human Immunodeficiency Virus (HIV) (AIDS) Infection

RECOGNITION OF CAUSE OF INFECTION	RESULTS OF CARE PROGRAM	GUIDES FOR ACTION
1. Transmission of infectious material: HIV-infected blood or blood-tinged body fluids.	1. Current infection control practices will be used in all instances to prevent contact with blood or with any body fluids or drainage.	1. Gloves will be worn at all times to prevent contact with infectious material.
2. Laboratory report of positive culture for disease process. (Dissemination of HIV testing results may be illegal in some states.)	2. Information will be given to patient and personnel, and patient care practices will show consistent use of methods of control transmission of HIV.	2. Masks may be worn if aerosols are possible during suction procedures. Goggles may be used to protect eyes.
3. Signs and symptoms: ☐ Low grade fever (> 100° F, intermittent or continuous for at least 3 mos.) ☐ Lymph node enlargement and tenderness ☐ Weight loss ☐ Diarrhea ☐ Thrush ☐ Presence of opportunistic infection ☐ Dry non-productive cough ☐ Drenching night sweats	3. Current cost-effective infection control measures will be demonstrated daily in patient care practices.	3. Soiled linen should be separated and labeled. Soiled dressings should be placed in plastic or paper bag, tied or sealed, and placed in trash.
4. HIV virus classification system: ☐ Grp I Acute infection ☐ Grp II Asymptomatic infection (some states require a patient release to report this category to the local health dept.)		4. Instruction concerning current methods of prevention of transmission of HIV will be given in regular sessions for all personnel and interested patients and their families.

- ☐ Grp III Persistent generalized
  lymphadenopathy
- ☐ Grp IV Other disease
  - ☐ Subgrp A Constitutional disease
  - ☐ Subgrp B Neurological disease
  - ☐ Subgrp C Secondary infectious
    diseases
    - ☐ Category C1 Specified
      secondary infectious disease
      listed in the CDC surveillance
      definition for AIDS
    - ☐ Category C2 Other specified
      secondary infectious diseases
  - ☐ Subgrp D Secondary cancers
  - ☐ Subgrp E Other conditions

Cost-Effective Measures for HIV (AIDS)-Infected Patient

In HIV (AIDS) infections, the infective material is blood, bloody feces, bloody sputum, or any body fluid containing blood.

The consistent application of preventive techniques to control the virus in any setting will result in the following:

1. Reduced incidence of infection.
2. Reduced health care cost for facility or patient and family.
3. Reduced risk of malpractice suits.
4. Reduced risk for the community.

When the HIV (AIDS)-infected patient is hospitalized, the following guides must be used:

1. Thorough handwashing using friction and soap under running water.
2. Wear gloves for any procedure involving contact with infected blood or body fluids.
3. Wear masks if suctioning or coughing of bloody sputum by patient is likely to produce a projectile spray. Goggles may be used to protect eyes.
4. Clean soiled areas with bleach solution (dilute 1:10 with water). Solution can be used to clean soiled equipment, floors, or areas soiled with infected blood. SOLUTION MUST BE MIXED DAILY.

When the HIV (AIDS)-infected patient is cared for at home, contact with blood or body secretions or excretions must be prevented and gloves should be worn. If gloves are unavailable, thorough handwashing must be done immediately after contact with infective material or contaminated surfaces. Instruct family to use dilute bleach solution on surfaces and equipment. Linen may be washed in regular washing machine with hot water, soap or detergent, and 2 cups of household bleach.

GASTROINTESTINAL SYSTEM
Guide to Control Infections

The gastrointestinal system includes the esophagus, the stomach, the jejunum, the upper and lower ileum, and the large intestine. The normal flora in this system is protective to the normal host, but in immunosuppressed hosts these organisms can be sources of infection in their normal area.

Trauma, surgery, fistulas, or other disruptions can allow gastrointestinal organisms into the blood, causing infections in other body sites. The physical health of the host and the medical treatment regimen (e.g., antibiotics) and procedures will have a bearing on the level of infection, if it occurs.

IN THE GASTROINTESTINAL SYSTEM, THE FECES OR BOWEL DRAINAGE IS THE INFECTIVE MATERIAL.

HANDWASHING IS ESSENTIAL:
- *Before and after the care of each patient.*
- *Before and after changing any dressing on any area of the gastrointestinal system.*
- *Before and after the administration of gastric tube feedings, or changing of gastric tube.*
- *Before and after any procedures involving contact with intestinal drainage.*

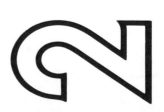

NOTES

2

Gastrointestinal System

SITE	ORGANISMS	TYPE OF STAIN	RELATED DISEASES	SIGNS AND SYMPTOMS
Esophagus	Very low numbers			
Stomach	With chronic use of antacids or if ulcers are present, the stomach may be colonized with microorganisms			
Jejunum	*Lactobacillus* sp	GP	Endocarditis (rare)	—
	Enterococcus sp (upper jejunum)	GP	—	—
	Streptococcus faecalis	GP	Endocarditis	—
	Bacteroides and *Clostridium* sp	GN	Peritonitis, abscess, enteritis, pseudomembranous enterocolitis, food poisoning	Pain, fever, nausea, vomiting, cramps, diarrhea
	Enterobacteriaceae	GN	Abscess, bacteremia	Pain, fever
	Mycobacterium sp	AF	Enteric fever	Pain, fever, nausea, vomiting, cramps, diarrhea
	Staphylococcus aureus	GP	Endocarditis	Pain, fever
Large intestine	More than 100 organisms are considered "normal" and are found in fecal smears and cultures			

Organism	Gram	Condition	Symptoms
Acinetobacter sp	GN	Postsurgical complications and infections in immunosuppressed hosts	General malaise, nausea, diarrhea, distention, pain
Clostridium sp	GP	Gallbladder inflammation	Nausea, vomiting, right quadrant pain, fever
C. perfringens	GP	Food poisoning	Nausea, vomiting, diarrhea, cramps
Enterococcus sp	GP	Peritonitis, abscess, UTI	Pain, fever, distention
Eubacterium sp	GP	—	—
Peptococcus sp	GP	Abscess	Nausea, vomiting, pain, fever, distention
Peptostreptococcus sp	GP	Abscess	As above
Streptococcus sp	GP	Abscess	As above
Staphylococcus sp	GP	Abscess	As above

SAMPLE AND INSTRUCTIONS FOR
CHARTS FOR HOSPITAL, HOME, OFFICE, AND OUTPATIENT CLINIC

Charts for Hospital, Home, Office, and Outpatient Clinic

DISEASE SPECIFIC CODES

ALL	At all times	SL	If soiling likely
D	Desirable, but optional	SUS	If susceptible
PH	Poor hygiene	WC	With contact

DISEASE	CATEGORY SPECIFIC		DISEASE SPECIFIC						
	Type	Duration	Handwashing—Thorough Rubbing, Lather, Rinsing	Private Room Needed	Masks	Gowns	Gloves	Linen—If Soiled, separate	Containers for Body Fluids; Precautions if Contaminated
Common cold									
Adults	–	–	ALL	–	–	–	–	–	–
Infants and children	CI	DI	ALL	ALL	SL	SL	–	–	–

HOW TO READ THIS CHART			CATEGORY SPECIFIC CODES	
Steps	**Example**		**Type**	**Duration**
1. Locate infection or disease; read from left to right.	Read first row across as: **Common cold in adults** requires *no* special precautions or supplies; *handwashing* is required to prevent transmission.		**AFB** Tuberculosis (AFB) isolation	**CN** Off antibiotics; culture negative
2. **Type** indicates *Category Specific* control measures.			**B/BF** Blood/body fluid precautions	**DH** Duration of hospitalization
3. **Duration** signifies length of time to use *Category Specific* control measures.	Read second row across as: **Common cold in infants and children** can require *contact isolation* for duration of infection; *handwashing* is required to prevent transmission; *private room and gloves* are recommended.		**CI** Contact isolation	**DI** Duration of illness/drainage
				U-a Until 24 hours after therapy begins
4. Use legend in upper left-hand corner to interpret codes in *Disease Specific* columns.			**D/S** Drainage/ secretion precautions	**U-b** Until 2 weeks after therapy begins or until sputa negative
				U-c For 9 days after swelling
5. Column headings in the *Disease Specific* section indicate procedures, patient area, and supplies to be used with *Disease Specific* control measures.			**EP** Enteric precautions	**U-d** For 7 days after rash or swelling or onset of infection
			RI Respiratory precautions	**U-e** For 3 days after therapy begins
				U-f For 4 days after rash begins; if immunosuppressed, use DI
			SI Strict isolation	**U-g** Until HBsAg (hepatitis B surface antigen) is negative
				U-h For 48 hours after effective therapy begins

2

Charts for Hospital, Home, Office, and Outpatient Clinic

DISEASE SPECIFIC CODES

ALL At all times
D   Desirable, but optional
PH   Poor hygiene

SL   If soiling likely
SUS If susceptible
WC   With contact

DISEASE	CATEGORY SPECIFIC		Handwashing, Thorough rubbing, Lather, rinsing	Private Room Needed	DISEASE SPECIFIC				
	Type	Duration			Masks	Gowns	Gloves	Linen—if soiled, separate	Containers for Body Fluids: Precautions if Contaminated
Acquired immunodeficiency syndrome (AIDS)[1]	B/BF	DI	ALL	PH	–	SL	WC	ALL	ALL
Amebiasis (dysentery)	EP	DI	ALL	PH	–	SL	WC	ALL	D
Bacillary dysentery (shigellosis)	E	U-e	ALL	PH	–	SL	WC	ALL	–
Botulism—any type	–	–	ALL	–	–	–	–	–	–
Campylobacter gastroenteritis	EP	DI	ALL	PH	–	SL	WC	ALL	D
Cholera	EP	DI	ALL	PH	–	SL	WC	ALL	D
Coxsackie virus disease[2]	EP	DI	ALL	PH	–	SL	WC	ALL	D
Diarrhea (acute infective etiology suspect; see Gastroenteritis)	EP	DI	ALL	PH	–	SL	WC	ALL	D
Echovirus disease[2]	EP	U-d	ALL	PH	–	SL	WC	ALL	D

Condition									
Encephalitis/encephalomyelitis (etiology unknown; infection suspect)[3]	EP	DI/U-d	ALL	PH	–	SL	WC	ALL	D
Enterobiasis (pinworm, oxyuriasis)	–	ALL	–	–	–	–	–	–	–
Enterocolitis (also necrotizing enterocolitis)									
Clostridium difficile	EP	DI	ALL	PH	–	SL	WC	ALL	D
Staphylococcus	EP	DI	ALL	PH	–	SL	WC	ALL	D
Enteroviral disease	EP	DI	ALL	PH	–	SL	WC	ALL	D
Escherichia coli gastroenteritis (enteropathic, enterotoxic, or enteroinvasive)	EP	DI	ALL	PH	–	SL	WC	ALL	D
Food poisoning									
Salmonellosis	EP	DI	ALL	PH	–	SL	WC	ALL	D
Staphylococcus	–	–	ALL	–	–	–	–	–	–
Gastroenteritis									
Campylobacter sp	EP	–	ALL	PH	–	SL	WC	ALL	D
Clostridium difficile	EP	–	ALL	PH	–	SL	WC	ALL	D
Cryptosporidium sp	EP	–	ALL	PH	–	SL	WC	ALL	D

1. Feces may contain blood; use gloves when contact with feces may occur.
2. Respiratory secretions are infective.
3. Likely causes are arthropod-borne virus and enterovirus.

continued

2

Charts for Hospital, Home, Office, and Outpatient Clinic *continued*

DISEASE SPECIFIC CODES

ALL	At all times
D	Desirable, but optional
PH	Poor hygiene
SL	If soiling likely
SUS	If susceptible
WC	With contact

DISEASE	CATEGORY SPECIFIC		Handwashing—Thorough rubbing, Lather, Rinsing	DISEASE SPECIFIC						
	Type	Duration		Private Room Needed	Masks	Gowns	Gloves	Linen—if Soiled, separate	Containers for Body Fluids; Precautions if Contaminated
Gastroenteritis *continued*									
Dientamoeba fragilis	EP	DI	ALL	PH	–	SL	WC	ALL	D
Escherichia coli (enterotoxic, enteropathic, or invasive)	EP	DI	ALL	PH	–	SL	WC	ALL	D
Giardia lamblia (giardiasis)	EP	DI	ALL	PH	–	SL	WC	ALL	D
Norwalk agent	EP	DI	ALL	PH	–	SL	WC	ALL	D
Rotavirus	EP	U-d	ALL	PH	–	SL	WC	ALL	D
Salmonella sp	EP	DI	ALL	PH	–	SL	WC	ALL	D
Shigella sp (includes bacillary dysentery)	EP	CN×3	ALL	PH	–	SL	WC	ALL	D
Streptococcus group B—in neonates[1]	–	–	ALL	–	–	–	–	–	–

Unknown etiology	EP	DI	ALL	PH	-	SL	WC	ALL	D
Vibrio parahaemolyticus	EP	DI	ALL	PH	-	SL	WC	ALL	D
Viral	EP	DI	ALL	PH	-	SL	WC	ALL	D
Yersinia enterolitica	EP	DI	ALL	PH	-	SL	WC	ALL	D
Hand, foot, and mouth disease	EP	U-d	ALL	PH	-	SL	WC	ALL	D
Hepatitis—viral, type A infectious	EP	U-d	ALL	PH	-	SL	WC	ALL	D
Herpangina	EP	U-d	ALL	PH	-	SL	WC	ALL	D
Meningitis—aseptic									
Nonbacterial or viral; see specific etiologies	EP	U-d	ALL	PH	-	SL	WC	ALL	D
Bacterial, gram-negative, in neonates[1]	-	-	ALL	-	-	-	-	-	-
Multiply resistant organisms—infection or colonization									
Gastrointestinal	CI	CN	ALL	-	-	SL	WC	ALL	D
Skin wound, burn[2]	CI	CN	ALL	-	-	SL	WC	ALL	D
Pleurodynia	EP	U-d	ALL	PH	-	SL	WC	ALL	D
Poliomyelitis	EP	U-d	ALL	PH	-	SL	WC	ALL	D
Rotavirus (gastroenteritis)	EP	U-d	ALL	PH	-	SL	WC	ALL	D

1. Feces may be infective In nurseries cohort Ill and colonized infants.
2. Feces may be infective

continued

2

Charts for Hospital, Home, Office, and Outpatient Clinic *continued*

DISEASE SPECIFIC CODES

ALL At all times	**SL** If soiling likely
D Desirable, but optional	**SUS** If susceptible
PH Poor hygiene	**WC** With contact

DISEASE	CATEGORY SPECIFIC		DISEASE SPECIFIC						
	Type	Duration	Handwashing—Thorough rubbing, Lather, Rinsing	Private Room Needed	Masks	Gowns	Gloves	Linen—if Soiled, separate	Containers for Body Fluids: Precautions if Contaminated
Strongyloidiasis[1]	-	-	ALL	-	-	-	-	-	-
Tapeworm disease[1]									
Vibrio–parahaemolyticus gastroenteritis	EP	DI	ALL	PH	-	SL	WC	ALL	D
Viral diseases, as pericarditis, myocarditis, or meningitis[2]	EP	U-d	ALL	PH	-	SL	WC	ALL	D

1. Feces may be infective.
2. Respiratory secretions as well as feces may be infective.

Sample Nursing Care Guide

RECOGNITION OF CAUSE OF INFECTION	RESULTS OF CARE PROGRAM	GUIDES FOR ACTION
1. Transmission of infectious material: gastrointestinal drainage, feces.	1. Patient will not become dehydrated.	1. Fluid will be encouraged within the limits of patient's intake requirements or limitations.
2. Laboratory report of positive culture for disease process.	2. Nausea, vomiting, and diarrhea will be controlled.	2. IV fluids will be monitored q. shift.
3. Signs and symptoms. ☐ fever ☐ pain ☐ nausea and vomiting ☐ diarrhea ☐ cramps ☐ dehydration	3. Infectious material will be handled and disposed of properly to prevent transmission.	3. Medications will be administered as prescribed for nausea, vomiting, or diarrhea.
	4. Patient and care givers in hospital or home will demonstrate appropriate control measures for gastrointestinal drainage and feces.	4. Good handwashing technique will be used at all times.
4. Knowledge deficit of patient or care givers in home or hospital regarding method of infection transmission.	5. Current cost-effective infection control measures will be demonstrated daily in patient care.	5. Supplies and equipment will be cleaned and disinfected or sterilized between patients.
		6. Feces and GI drainage will be disposed of in toilet.

2

Sample Discharge Guide

GENERAL POINTS FOR DISCHARGE	GUIDE FOR CARE IN A CLINIC OR NON-HOSPITAL SETTING	GUIDE FOR CARE IN HOME	GUIDE FOR CARE IN SNF
Information to transmit to anyone receiving a patient with a gastrointestinal infection:	1. Use thorough handwashing before and after all patient care.	1. Use thorough handwashing before and after taking care of patient.	1. Use thorough handwashing before and after all patient care.
1. Identify the source of infection: gastrointestinal drainage, feces.	2. Use gloves if there is a possibility of CONTACT with feces or any other intestinal drainage.	2. Use gloves if contact with infective material is possible. *Note:* Gloves are an expensive item for use in the home by family members. Handwashing if done conscientiously has proved to be sufficient in the home.	2. Use gloves if there is a possibility of CONTACT with feces or bowel drainage.
2. Describe the method of transmission and the infection control measures necessary to prevent contact with infectious material.	3. Use gowns to protect clothing if there is a possibility of any soiling by drainage.		3. Use gowns if soiling is likely.
			4. No special precautions necessary for linens or dishes.
3. Review all medications prescribed.	4. Dispose of liquid or solid body wastes in regular toilet.	3. No special precautions are necessary for linens or dishes.	5. Dispose of liquid or solid body wastes in regular toilet.
4. Notify any agency or transport personnel of special precautions needed to prevent contact with infectious material.	5. Place soiled diapers (infant/adult) in plastic or heavy paper bag, tie or seal and place in trash.	4. Use regular toilet for disposal of liquid or solid body waste.	6. Place soiled diapers in a plastic or heavy paper bag, tie or seal, and place in trash.
5. Inform public health department if the infection is reportable.	6. Clean surfaces, if soiling occurs, with bleach solution diluted 1:10 with water.	5. Dispose of soiled diapers (infant/adult) in plastic or heavy paper bag, tie or seal and place in trash.	7. If spills or soiling occurs, clean surfaces with bleach solution diluted 1:10 with water.
		6. Clean surfaces, if spills or soiling occurs, with bleach solution diluted 1:10 with water.	

Cost-Effective Measures

The use of proven infection control measures, not rituals, to care for patients with communicable diseases is cost effective. When nursing consistently applies these measures in the health care setting, they reduce infections and death, reduce costs for the facility and patient, reduce potential malpractice suits, facilitate the accreditation process, and strengthen the infection control program as a whole.

When the patient is hospitalized, the following guidelines must be used:

1. Use good handwashing technique at all times.
2. Recognize cases of gastroenteritis promptly.
3. Initiate appropriate isolation techniques to prevent cross-contamination.
4. Screen patients for diarrheal illness on admission, especially maternity patients. Use isolation precautions for newborns to prevent cross-contamination.

When the patient is cared for at home, optimum clean techniques are acceptable. The simplest methods to keep the home clean, orderly, and safe are the most practical and cost-effective methods. Rarely will it be necessary to take the "sterile" emphasis into the home. The patient will be returning to a known environment where there will be few if any unusual organisms. Handwashing and NO TOUCH TECHNIQUE are the most important factors to emphasize in the home for wound care and drainage secretion and excretion control. These optimum clean techniques will prevent transmission of infective material.

GENITOURINARY SYSTEM
Guide to Control Infections

The genitourinary system is a dual system composed of (1) the external genitalia and organs necessary to sexual function and (2) the urinary system, which includes the bladder and kidneys.

The bladder and kidneys are sterile, as is the proximal length of the urethra as it enters the bladder. The outer opening and a short length of the urethra are colonized with normal flora. These organisms can become pathogenic if displaced into the bladder, kidneys, prostate, or testicular sac.

Infections of the urinary tract and bladder are the most common nosocomial and community-acquired infections. A urinary tract infection (UTI) can cause bacteremia, septicemia, and death. Endogenous UTIs can be caused by the displacement of normal flora. Exogenous UTIs are caused by unsterile or unclean procedures and unwashed hands. Host factors that predispose patients to UTI include age, physical health, sex, and the postpartum condition.

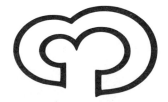

IN THE GENITOURINARY SYSTEM, THE URINE AND GENITAL SECRETIONS ARE THE SOURCES OF INFECTION.

HANDWASHING IS ESSENTIAL:

- *Before and after the care of each patient.*
- *Before and after performing any genital or perineal care.*
- *Before and after preparation for ANY sterile procedure such as instrumentation or catheterization of the urethra or bladder.*
- *Before and after handling urine or genital secretions.*

Genitourinary System

SITE	ORGANISMS	TYPE STAIN	RELATED DISEASES	SIGNS AND SYMPTOMS
Bladder, kidneys, prostate, testicles, urethra	None			
Penis, vagina, cervix, anterior urethra, external genitals	*Acinetobacter*	GN	Urethritis	Itch, inflammation, purulence
	Candida sp	Yeast	Candidiasis	Itch, heavy discharge
	Clostridium sp	GP	Postoperative complications	Purulence, fever, distention
	Corynebacterium sp	GN	Pyelonephritis, cystitis, bacteremia	Flank pain, anuria, Incontinence; blood culture positive
	Gardnerella sp	GN	Vaginitis	Now in venereal classification
	Lactobacillus sp	GP	Rarely postoperative complications	Bacteremia
	Peptococcus sp	GN	Postpartum complications	Purulence, foul odor, fever
	Bacteroides sp	GP		
	Staphylococcus sp	GP	Toxic shock	Severe prostration to coma
	S. aureus	GP	Urethritis	Itch, purulence
	All other areas not listed	As nec. for ID	UTI, vaginitis, epididymitis, urethritis, anal fistula, perineal abscess	Bacteruria, pyuria, hematuria, frequency, burning, fever, foul odor to urine or secretions, dysuria, lesions

3

NOTES

SAMPLE AND INSTRUCTIONS FOR
CHARTS FOR HOSPITAL, HOME, OFFICE, AND OUTPATIENT CLINIC

Charts for Hospital, Home, Office, and Outpatient Clinic

DISEASE SPECIFIC CODES

ALL	At all times	**SL**	If soiling likely
D	Desirable, but optional	**SUS**	If susceptible
PH	Poor hygiene	**WC**	With contact

DISEASE	CATEGORY SPECIFIC		DISEASE SPECIFIC					
	Type	Duration	Handwashing, Thorough Rubbing—Lather, Rinsing	Private Room Needed	Masks	Gowns	Gloves	Linen—if Soiled, separate	Containers for Body Fluids; Precautions if Contaminated
Common cold									
Adults	-	-	ALL	-	-	-	-	-	-
Infants and children	CI	DI	ALL	ALL	-	SL	-	-	-

HOW TO READ THIS CHART			CATEGORY SPECIFIC CODES	
Steps	Example	Type		Duration
1. Locate infection or disease; read from left to right.	Read first row across as: **Common cold in adults** *requires no special* precautions or supplies; *handwashing* is required to prevent transmission.	AFB	Tuberculosis (AFB) isolation	CN Off antibiotics; culture negative
2. **Type** indicates *Category Specific* control measures.		B/BF	Blood/body fluid precautions	DH Duration of hospitalization
3. **Duration** signifies length of time to use *Category Specific* control measures.	Read second row across as: **Common cold in infants and children** can require *contact isolation* for duration of infection; *handwashing* is required to prevent transmission; *private room and gloves* are recommended.	CI	Contact isolation	DI Duration of illness/drainage
4. Use legend in upper left-hand corner to interpret codes in *Disease Specific* columns.		D/S	Drainage/ secretion precautions	U-a Until 24 hours after therapy begins
				U-b Until 2 weeks after therapy begins or until sputa negative
		EP	Enteric precautions	U-c For 9 days after swelling
				U-d For 7 days after rash or swelling or onset of infection
5. Column headings in the *Disease Specific* section indicate procedures, patient area, and supplies to be used with *Disease Specific* control measures.		RI	Respiratory precautions	U-e For 3 days after therapy begins
		SI	Strict isolation	U-f For 4 days after rash begins; if immunosuppressed, use DI
				U-g Until HBsAg (hepatitis B surface antigen) is negative
				U-h For 48 hours after effective therapy begins

3

Charts for Hospital, Home, Office, and Outpatient Clinic

DISEASE SPECIFIC CODES

ALL At all times
D Desirable, but optional
PH Poor hygiene

SL If soiling likely
SUS If susceptible
WC With contact

DISEASE	CATEGORY SPECIFIC				DISEASE SPECIFIC				
	Type	Duration	Handwashing—Thorough Rubbing, Lather, rinsing	Private Room Needed	Masks	Gowns	Gloves	Linen—if soiled, separate	Containers for Body Fluids, precautions if Contaminated
Chlamydia trachomatis (genital)	D/S	DI	ALL	–	–	–	WC	–	–
Congenital rubella[1,2]	CI	DI	ALL	ALL	–	SL	WC	ALL	ALL
Endometritis									
Group A *Streptococcus*	CI	U-a	ALL	PH	–	SL	WC	ALL	ALL
Other	D/S	DI	ALL	–	–	SL	WC	ALL	ALL
Leptospirosis (blood and urine infections)	B/BF	DH	ALL	–	–	–	WC	–	ALL
Multiply resistant organisms									
Urine[3]	CI	CN	ALL	ALL	–	–	WC	ALL	ALL
Feces	CI	CN	ALL	ALL	–	SL	WC	ALL	ALL

	CI	U-a	ALL	PH		SL	WC	ALL	ALL
Puerperal sepsis (endometritis)	D/S	DI	ALL	-	-	SL	WC	ALL	-
Toxic shock syndrome									
Syphilis with lesions (includes congenital, primary, secondary)	B/BF D/S	U-a	ALL	-	-	-	D	-	-

1. Isolation precautions for first year after birth, unless nasopharyngeal and urine cultures are negative for rubella virus after 3 months.
2. Pregnant personnel may need counseling. Susceptibles should stay out of room. See CDC *Guidelines for Infection Control for Hospital Personnel.*
3. Patients with Foley catheters may be cohorted if organism is the same.

Sample Nursing Care Guide

RECOGNITION OF CAUSE OF INFECTION	RESULTS OF CARE PROGRAM	GUIDES FOR ACTION
1. Transmission of infective material: urine or genital secretions.	1. Infective material—urine or genital secretions—will be handled and disposed of properly to prevent transmission.	1. Urine-measuring containers should be issued to individual patients including those not infected.
2. Laboratory report of positive culture for disease process.	2. Soiled peripads or diapers will be handled and disposed of properly to prevent transmission.	2. Cohort or separate those with infections; or place in rooms with patients who do not have catheters or invasive devices.
3. Signs and symptoms: ☐ fever ☐ burning on urination ☐ frequency ☐ flank pain ☐ foul odor ☐ distention ☐ itch ☐ inflammation ☐ purulent or heavy discharge ☐ hematuria ☐ dysuria ☐ bacteriuria	3. Susceptible personnel will be notified of possible risk (i.e., pregnant or at risk because of non-immune status).	3. Thorough handwashing before and after any patient care.
	4. Current cost-effective measures will be demonstrated daily in patient care practices.	4. Use of gloves if CONTACT with genitourinary secretions or drainage is possible.
		5. Use regular toilet for body wastes.
4. Knowledge deficit of patient or care givers in any setting, regarding method of transmission of infection.		6. Dispose of soiled peripads in plastic or heavy paper bags, tie or seal, and place in trash.
		7. Notification of pregnant, or other susceptible personnel at risk for infection (e.g., cytomegalovirus [CMV] infection or congenital rubella).

Sample Discharge Guide

GENERAL POINTS FOR DISCHARGE	GUIDE FOR CARE IN A CLINIC OR NON-HOSPITAL SETTING	GUIDE FOR CARE IN HOME	GUIDE FOR CARE IN SNF
Information to transmit to anyone receiving a patient with a genitourinary infection.	1. Use thorough handwashing before and after all patient care.	1. Use thorough handwashing before and after taking care of patient.	1. Use thorough handwashing before and after all patient care.
1. Identify the source of infection: urogenital secretions.	2. Use gloves when there is a possibility of CONTACT with urine or genital secretions.	2. Use gloves if contact with infective material is possible. Note: Gloves are an expensive item for use in the home by family members. Handwashing if done conscientiously has proved to be sufficient in the home setting.	2. Use gloves if there is a possibility of CONTACT with urine or genital secretions.
2. Describe method of transmission and the infection control measures necessary to prevent contact with infective material.	3. Use gowns if soiling is likely.		3. Use gown if soiling is likely.
	4. Use regular toilet for disposal of liquid or solid body wastes.	3. No special precautions necessary for linens or dishes.	4. No special precautions necessary for linens or dishes.
3. Review all medication prescribed. Note: Gyn infections may be contagious until therapy is started.	5. Use plastic or heavy paper bag for soiled perineal pads. Tie or seal bag and place in trash.	4. Use regular toilet to dispose of liquid or solid body wastes. Note: Toilet seats are a rare source of infection.	5. Place soiled perineal pads in plastic or heavy paper bag, tie or seal, and place in trash.
	6. Clean surfaces promptly if any spills or soiling occurs. Use approved disinfectant.	5. Clean surfaces promptly if spills or soiling occurs; use bleach solution diluted 1:10 with water.	6. Use regular toilet for the disposal of liquid or solid body wastes.
4. Notify any agency or transport personnel of special procedures needed to prevent contact with infectious material.	7. Caution pregnant personnel regarding care of these patients if congenital rubella or cytomegalovirus is the cause of infection.	6. Vaccinate siblings, or family members if appropriate, as with congenital rubella.	7. If spills or soiling occurs, clean surfaces with approved disinfectant.
5. Inform public health department if infection is reportable.			8. Caution pregnant personnel regarding care of these patients if congenital rubella or cytomegalovirus is the cause of the infection.

Cost-Effective Measures

The use of proven infection control measures, not rituals, to care for patients with communicable diseases is cost effective. When nursing consistently applies these measures in the health care setting, they reduce infections and death, reduce costs for the facility or patients, reduce potential malpractice suits, facilitate the accreditation process, and strengthen the infection control program as a whole.

When the patient is hospitalized, the following guidelines must be used:

1. Use good handwashing technique at all times.
2. Catheterize only when necessary; leave catheter in place only as long as necessary.
3. Wash hands *before and after* any manipulation of catheter site or apparatus. Use gloves if soiling is likely.
4. Insert catheter using aseptic technique and sterile equipment.
5. Secure catheter properly.
6. Maintain closed sterile drainage.
7. Obtain urine samples with sterile technique.
8. Maintain unobstructed urine flow:
   ☐ No kinks in catheter or collecting tube.
   ☐ Separate collecting containers for each patient.
   ☐ Poorly functioning or obstructed catheters should be irrigated or, if necessary, replaced.
   ☐ Keep collecting bags below level of bladder.
9. Patients with indwelling catheters should be separated.

When the patient is cared for at home, optimum clean techniques are acceptable. The simplest methods to keep the home clean, orderly, and safe are the most practical and cost-effective methods. Rarely will it be necessary to take the "sterile" emphasis into the home. The patient will be returning to a known environment where there will be few if any unusual organisms. Handwashing and NO TOUCH TECHNIQUE are the most important factors to emphasize in the home for wound care and drainage secretion or excretion control. These optimum clean techniques will prevent transmission of infective material.

3

THE INTEGUMENTARY SYSTEM: SKIN AND UNDERLYING TISSUE
Guide to Control Infections

This system is the *first* line of defense against invasion of microorganisms into all body systems. Many organisms are present on the skin. The presence of these organisms does not mean *infection*; however, their presence does indicate *colonization*. The risk of infection is directly related to the length of time any type of skin damage persists. Displacement of surface organisms into dermal or fascial tissue magnifies the risk of infection for the whole system. The repair and healing of breaks in the skin are related to host factors such as physical health, age, circulatory problems, and nutrition. Any wound, whether surgical or traumatic, or skin break at any stage creates the potential risk of infection.

IN THE INTEGUMENTARY SYSTEM, PUS OR EXUDATE FROM LESIONS IS THE INFECTIVE MATERIAL.

HANDWASHING IS ESSENTIAL:
- *Before and after the care of each patient.*
- *Before and after any form of wound care.*

The Integumentary System

SITE	ORGANISMS	TYPE STAIN	RELATED DISEASES	SIGNS AND SYMPTOMS
Skin surface	*Staphylococcus epidermidis*	GP	Acne, endocarditis, complications in heart surgery, bacteremias	Pus, positive blood cultures, systemic signs (e.g., fever, malaise, coma)
	S. aureus	GP	Bacteremia, commonly associated with total parenteral nutrition (TPN) site infections	Pus, positive cultures; systemic signs (e.g. fever, malaise, coma)
	Corynebacterium sp (diphtheroid)	GP	Pustules, furuncles, boils, impetigo, endocarditis	Cellulitis without pus, pus, inflamed lumps, systemic signs, fatigue
	Propionibacterium acnes	GP	Acne, pimples, bacterial endocarditis	Local pus pockets, systemic signs (e.g., fever, fatigue, malaise)
	Pityrospcrum ovale	Yeast	Paronychia nail infection, itchy patches, athlete's foot	Black nails, loss of nails: dry, red skin patch; moist, weepy skin
	Candida albicans	Yeast		
	Dermatophytes	Fungus-specific	Athlete's foot, nail infections, skin infections, generalized infection	As above

SAMPLE AND INSTRUCTIONS FOR
CHARTS FOR HOSPITAL, HOME, OFFICE, AND OUTPATIENT CLINIC

Charts for Hospital, Home, Office, and Outpatient Clinic

DISEASE SPECIFIC CODES

ALL	At all times	**SL**	If soiling likely
D	Desirable, but optional	**SUS**	If susceptible
PH	Poor hygiene	**WC**	With contact

DISEASE	CATEGORY SPECIFIC		DISEASE SPECIFIC						
	Type	Duration	Handwashing, Thorough rubbing, Lather, Rinsing	Private Room Needed	Masks	Gowns	Gloves	Linen—if Soiled, separate	Containers for Body Fluids; precautions if Contaminated
Common cold									
Adults	–	–	ALL	–	–	–	–	–	–
Infants and children	CI	DI	ALL	ALL	–	SL	–	–	–

HOW TO READ THIS CHART			CATEGORY SPECIFIC CODES	
Steps	Example		Type	Duration
1. Locate infection or disease; read from left to right.	Read first row across as: **Common cold in adults** *requires no special precautions or supplies; handwashing is required to prevent transmission.*	**AFB** Tuberculosis (AFB) isolation	**CN** Off antibiotics; culture negative
2. **Type** indicates *Category Specific* control measures.			**DH** Duration of hospitalization
		B/BF Blood/body fluid precautions	**DI** Duration of illness/drainage
3. **Duration** signifies length of time to use *Category Specific* control measures.	Read second row across as: **Common cold in infants and children** can require *contact isolation* for duration of infection; *handwashing is required to prevent transmission; private room and gloves are recommended.*		**U-a** Until 24 hours after therapy begins
		CI Contact isolation	**U-b** Until 2 weeks after therapy begins or until sputa negative
4. Use legend in upper left-hand corner to interpret codes in *Disease Specific* columns.			**U-c** For 9 days after swelling
		D/S Drainage/ secretion precautions	**U-d** For 7 days after rash or swelling or onset of infection
		EP Enteric precautions	**U-e** For 3 days after therapy begins
5. Column headings in the *Disease Specific* section indicate procedures, patient area, and supplies to be used with *Disease Specific* control measures.			**U-f** For 4 days after rash begins; if immunosuppressed, use DI
		RI Respiratory precautions	**U-g** Until HBsAg (hepatitis B surface antigen) is negative
		SI Strict isolation	**U-h** For 48 hours after effective therapy begins

4

57

Charts for Hospital, Home, Office, and Outpatient Clinic

DISEASE SPECIFIC CODES

ALL At all times
D Desirable, but optional
PH Poor hygiene
SL If soiling likely
SUS If susceptible
WC With contact

DISEASE	CATEGORY SPECIFIC				DISEASE SPECIFIC				
	Type	duration	Handwashing—Thorough rubbing, Lather, rinsing	Private Room Needed	Masks	Gowns	Gloves	Linen—if Soiled, separate	Containers for Body fluids; precautions if Contaminated
Abscess (etiology unknown)									
Draining, major wound[1]	CI	DI	ALL	ALL	–	SL	WC	ALL	D
Minor or limited wound	D/S	DI	ALL	–	–	SL	WC	ALL	–
Not draining	–	–	ALL	–	–	–	–	–	–
Actinomycosis—all lesions	–	–	ALL	–	–	–	–	–	–
Anthrax—cutaneous	D/S	DI	ALL	–	–	–	WC	ALL	–
Brucellosis—draining lesions	D/S	DI	ALL	–	–	SL	WC	ALL	–
Cellulitis									
Draining, limited or minor	D/S	DI	ALL	–	–	SL	WC	ALL	–

Intact skin	-	-	ALL	-	-	-	-	-	-
Chancroid (soft chancre)	-	-	ALL	-	-	-	-	-	-
Chickenpox (varicella)[2,3,4]	SI	-	ALL	D	SUS	ALL	ALL	ALL	ALL
Chlamydia trachomatis conjunctivitis	D/S	DI	ALL	-	-	-	WC	-	-
Conjunctivitis—gonococcal, in newborn[5]	CI	U-a	ALL	ALL	-	-	WC	-	-
Acute bacterial (pinkeye sore eye)	DS	DI	ALL	-	-	-	WC	-	-
Closed cavity infection—drainage limited or minor[6]	D/S	DI	ALL	-	-	SL	WC	ALL	-
Clostridium perfringens									
Gas gangrene	D/S	DI	ALL	-	-	SL	WC	ALL	-
Other	D/S	DI	ALL	-	-	SL	WC	ALL	-
Coccidioidomycosis—draining lesions[6]	-	-	ALL	-	-	-	-	-	-
Congenital rubella[4]	CI	DI	ALL	ALL	-	SL	WC	ALL	-

1. May cohort patients with same organism infecting wounds.
2. Until all lesions crusted.
3. If infection in the home, private room not needed.
4. Respiratory secretions are infective.
5. In gonococcal conjunctivitis infections in adults, handwashing is the only recommendation, unless hygiene is poor, when a private room may be desirable.
6. Drainage may be infective if spores are formed.

4

Charts for Hospital, Home, Office, and Outpatient Clinic *continued*

DISEASE SPECIFIC CODES

ALL At all times	**SL** If soiling likely
D Desirable, but optional	**SUS** If susceptible
PH Poor hygiene	**WC** With contact

DISEASE	CATEGORY SPECIFIC				DISEASE SPECIFIC				
	Type	Duration	Handwashing Thorough rubbing—Lather, rinsing	Private Room Needed	Masks	Gowns	Gloves	Linen—if Soiled, separate	Containers for Body fluids; precautions if Contaminated
Decubitus ulcer—infected									
Major, wound	CI	DI	ALL	ALL	–	SL	WC	ALL	–
Minor, limited	D/S	DI	ALL	–	–	SL	WC	ALL	–
Diphtheria—cutaneous	CI	CN	ALL	ALL	–	SL	WC	ALL	–
Eczema vaccinatum (vaccinia)	CI	DI	ALL	ALL	–	SL	WC	ALL	–
Furunculosis (staphylococcal)									
Newborns[1]	CI	DI	ALL	ALL	–	SL	WC	ALL	–
Others	D/S	DI	ALL	–	–	SL	WC	ALL	–
Gangrene due to any bacteria	D/S	DI	ALL	–	–	SL	WC	ALL	–

Gonococcal conjunctivitis									
Adult	D/S	U-a	ALL	-	-	-	WC	-	-
Newborns	CI	U-a	ALL	ALL	-	-	WC	ALL	-
German measles (rubella)[2]	CI	U-d	ALL	ALL	SUS	-	-	-	-
Herpes simplex									
Mucocutaneous, disseminated or primary; severe skin, oral, genital infection	CI	DI	ALL	ALL	-	SL	WC	ALL	D
Mucocutaneous, recurrent[1]	-	-	ALL	-	-	-	WC	-	D
Neonate[3]	CI	DI	ALL	ALL	-	SL	WC	ALL	D
Herpes zoster (varicella zoster)									
In immunocompromised host—disseminated	SI	DI	ALL	ALL	SUS	ALL	WC	ALL	ALL
In normal patient—localized (chickenpox)[4]	D/S	-	ALL	PH	-	-	WC	-	-
Impetigo	CI	U-a	ALL	PH	-	SL	WC	ALL	-
Keratoconjunctivitis—infective	D/S	DI	ALL	PH	-	-	WC	-	-

1. May be cohorted.
2. See also *Congenital rubella*.
3. The same precautions are indicated for infants delivered vaginally or by cesarean, if membranes ruptured 4 to 6 hours prior to delivery, if mother has active genital herpes. Risks may require the same precautions if membranes are unruptured.
4. Until all lesions crusted.

4

continued

Charts for Hospital, Home, Office, and Outpatient Clinic *continued*

DISEASE SPECIFIC CODES

ALL At all times	**SL** If soiling likely
D Desirable, but optional	**SUS** If susceptible
PH Poor hygiene	**WC** With contact

DISEASE	Type	Duration	Handwashing—Thorough Rubbing, Lather, Rinsing	Private Room Needed	Masks	Gowns	Gloves	Linen—if soiled, separate	Containers for Body Fluids; precautions if Contaminated
	CATEGORY SPECIFIC				DISEASE SPECIFIC				
Multiply resistant organisms									
Infection or colonization skin, wound, burn	CI	CN	ALL	ALL	-	SL	WC	ALL	ALL
Mycobacterium, atypical wound	D/S	DI	ALL	-	-	SL	WC	ALL	-
Nocardiosis—draining lesion	-	-	ALL	-	-	-	D	-	-
Pediculosis	CI	U-a	ALL	PH	-	WC	WC	ALL	-
Plague—bubonic	D/S	U-e	ALL	-	-	SL	WC	ALL	-
Ritter's disease (scalded skin syndrome, staphylococcal)[1]	CI	DI	ALL	ALL	-	SL	WC	ALL	D
Rubella (German measles)[2]	CI	U-d	ALL	ALL	SUS	-	-	-	-
Congenital	CI	DI	ALL	ALL	SUS	SL	WC	ALL	-

Scabies[3]	CI	DI	ALL	PH	–	WC	WC	ALL	–
Scaldec skin syndrome[1]	CI	DI	ALL	ALL	–	SL	WC	ALL	–
Smallpox[4]	SI	DI	ALL	ALL	ALL	ALL	ALL	ALL	ALL
Staphylococcal disease (skin, wound, or burn)									
Major as defined	CI	DI	ALL	ALL	–	SL	WC	ALL	D
Minor or limited	D/S	DI	ALL	–	–	SL	WC	ALL	D
Streptococcal disease									
Group A (skin, wound, burn)									
Major	CI	U-a	ALL	ALL	–	SL	WC	ALL	D
Minor	D/S	U-a	ALL	–	–	SL	WC	ALL	D
Group B (may be in feces)[5]	–	–	ALL	–	–	–	–	–	–

1. Infected and colonized patients may be cohorted.
2. Susceptibles should stay out of room. Pregnant employees may need counseling. See Rubella, in Respiratory System.
3. A mite infestation.
4. As long as smallpox vaccine is kept in laboratory stock, the potential for cases exists. Call State Health Department and CDC for help with case or suspected case.
5. During nursery outbreak of Streptococcus group B cohorting is recommended; use gowns and gloves.

continued

4

Charts for Hospital, Home, Office, and Outpatient Clinic *continued*

DISEASE SPECIFIC CODES

ALL At all times
D Desirable, but optional
PH Poor hygiene

SL If soiling likely
SUS If susceptible
WC With contact

DISEASE	CATEGORY SPECIFIC		Handwashing—Thorough rubbing, Lather, rinsing	Private Room Needed	DISEASE SPECIFIC			Linen—if Soiled, separate	Containers for Body Fluids, Precautions if Contaminated
	Type	Duration			Masks	Gowns	Gloves		
Syphilis, mucous membrane									
(Includes congenital, primary, and secondary)[1]	D/S & B/BF	U-a	ALL	–	–	–	D	–	–
Tertiary (no lesions)	–	–	ALL	–	–	–	–	–	–
Tuberculosis—extrapulmonary draining lesion (includes scrofula)[2]	D/S	DI	ALL	–	–	SL	WC	ALL	D
Tularemia—draining lesions	D/S	DI	ALL	–	–	SL	WC	ALL	D
Vaccinia at site	D/S	DI	ALL	–	–	SL	WC	–	D
Generalized, progressive eczema	CI	DI	ALL	ALL	–	SL	WC	ALL	D
Varicella (chickenpox)[3,4,5]	SI	–	ALL	SUS	ALL	ALL	ALL	ALL	ALL

Variola (smallpox)	SI	DI	ALL	ALL	ALL	ALL	ALL	ALL	ALL
Viral conjunctivitis—etiology unknown (acute, hemorrhagic, and swimming pool conjunctivitis)	D/S	DI	ALL	-	-	SL	WC	ALL	-
Wound infections									
Major	CI	DI	ALL	ALL	-	SL	WC	ALL	D
Minor or limited	D/S	DI	ALL	-	-	SL	WC	ALL	-
Zoster (Herpes)—all patients[3,6]	SI	-	ALL	ALL	SUS	ALL	ALL	ALL	ALL

1. Skin lesions and blood of primary and secondary syphilis are highly infective.
2. A private room is important for children.
3. Until all lesions crusted.
4. If infection in the home, private room not needed.
5. Respiratory secretions are infective.
6. See also *Herpes zoster*, normal patients or immunocompromised host.

65

4

Sample Nursing Care Guides

RECOGNITION OF CAUSE OF INFECTION	RESULTS OF CARE PROGRAM	GUIDES FOR ACTION
1. Transmission of infective material: pus or exudate from lesions or wounds.	1. Infectious material—pus or exudate from lesions—will be handled and disposed of properly to prevent transmission.	1. Laboratory culture and smears will regularly be reviewed and correlated with clinical signs by nursing.
2. Laboratory report of positive culture for infectious process.	2. Patient and care givers in home or hospital will demonstrate appropriate control measures for the care of wound and skin infections.	2. Handwashing will be done prior to all dressing changes. Use NO TOUCH TECHNIQUE.
3. Signs and symptoms: ☐ fever ☐ redness ☐ swelling ☐ heat ☐ pain ☐ purulent drainage ☐ cellulitis without pus ☐ malaise	3. Instruction will be given to update all personnel in the control measures necessary to prevent transmission of wound and skin infections.	3. All soiled dressings will be placed in bags, sealed or tied, and placed in trash.
	4. Removal of tape holding dressings will be done gently to prevent tearing skin.	4. In-service pertinent to the specific infection will be held in patient care areas in a timely manner.
4. Knowledge deficit by patient or care givers, in hospital or home, regarding transmission of infection.	5. Current cost-effective measures will be demonstrated daily in patient care practices.	5. Assess skin daily for abrasions. Tape will be removed without tearing. Limit taping on fragile skin.
5. Skin fragility due to aging, treatment modalities, disease process, chronic abuse of alcohol or drugs.		

Sample Discharge Guide

GENERAL POINTS FOR DISCHARGE	GUIDE FOR CARE IN A CLINIC OR NON-HOSPITAL SETTING	GUIDE FOR CARE IN HOME	GUIDE FOR CARE IN SNF
Information to transmit to anyone receiving a patient with a wound or skin infection	1. Use thorough hand-washing before and after all patient care.	1. Use thorough handwashing before and after taking care of patient.	1. Use thorough handwashing before and after all patient care.
1. Identify the source of infection: pus or exudate from lesions.	2. Use gloves if there is possibility of CONTACT with pus or lesion exudate.	2. Use gloves if contact with infectious material is possible. *Note:* Gloves are an expensive item for use in the home by family members. Handwashing if done conscientiously has proven to be sufficient in the home setting.	2. Use gloves if there is a possibility of CONTACT with pus or drainage.
2. Describe method of transmission and the infection control measures necessary to prevent contact with infective material.	3. Use gowns if there is extensive drainage and if soiling of clothing is likely.	3. Wash linens and dishes in usual manner.	3. Use gowns to protect clothing from wound drainage or pus.
3. Review all medications prescribed.	4. Handle dressings carefully. NO TOUCH TECHNIQUE is preferred.	4. Use apron or clean towel to cover clothing if drainage is excessive when doing dressing change.	4. Handle dressings carefully. Use NO TOUCH TECHNIQUE.
4. Describe dressing change method to use when caring for wound or lesions. NO TOUCH TECHNIQUE is preferred.	5. Place soiled dressings in plastic or heavy paper bag, seal or tie, and place in trash.	5. Handle dressings carefully. Use NO TOUCH TECHNIQUE.	5. Place soiled dressings in plastic or heavy paper bag, tie or seal, and place in trash.
5. Notify any agency or transport personnel of special procedures needed to prevent contact with infective material.	6. Clean surfaces promptly with an approved disinfectant if spills or soiling occurs.	6. Place soiled dressing in plastic or heavy paper bag, tie or seal, and dispose of in trash.	6. Remove tape carefully when removing dressings to prevent skin tearing.
6. Inform public health department if infection is reportable.		7. Protect skin from the trauma of tears when tape is removed or when the patient is turned or lifted with sheets.	7. Reposition patient carefully to prevent skin burns or shearing.
		8. Clean surfaces if spills or soiling occurs with bleach solution diluted 1:10 with water.	8. No special precautions are necessary for linens or dishes.
			9. Clean surfaces promptly with an approved disinfectant if spills or soiling occurs.

4

Cost-Effective Measures

The use of proven infection control measures, not rituals, to care for patients with communicable diseases is cost effective. When nursing consistently applies these measures in the health care setting they reduce infections and death, reduce costs for the facility or patient, reduce the potential for malpractice suits, facilitate the accreditation process, and strengthen the infection control program as a whole.

When the patient is hospitalized, the following guides must be used:

1. Use good handwashing techniques at all times.
2. Recognize instances of skin changes promptly.
3. Initiate measures to prevent skin trauma during patient care.
4. Obtain cultures of drainage to identify infective agent, if possible.

When the patient is cared for at home, optimum clean techniques are acceptable. The simplest methods to keep the home clean, orderly, and safe are the most practical and cost-effective methods. Rarely will it be necessary to take the ''sterile'' emphasis into the home. The patient will be returning to a known environment where there will be few if any unusual organisms. Handwashing and NO TOUCH TECHNIQUE are the most important factors to emphasize in the home for wound care and drainage secretion and excretion control. These optimum clean techniques will prevent transmission of infective material.

4

NOTES

MUSCULOSKELETAL SYSTEM
Guide to Control Infections

The musculoskeletal system is composed of all the bones, muscles and joints in the body. Several types of infections can affect this system, including osteomyelitis, septic (infectious) arthritis, and infections in or around skeletal prosthetic devices.

Osteomyelitis can affect all age groups and may be of long duration, from months to years. Generally, the sources of this infection are distant foci, such as the skin or urinary tract, or soft-tissue infections that develop in traumatic or surgical wounds. Usually, involved bones are the long bones, especially these of the lower extremities. Drug therapy is preferred over surgical intervention and is generally continued for 2 to 4 weeks. In chronic osteomyelitis, surgical debridement frequently is necessary.

Septic (infectious) arthritis can have tragic consequences for patients, including permanent loss of joint function, chronic osteomyelitis, or even death. Predisposing factors include prior joint diseases, endocarditis, serious underlying systemic disorders, and cytotoxic or immunosuppressive therapy. Systemic antibiotic therapy, along with synovial fluid aspirations, is the treatment of choice. Immobilization of the affected joint is also necessary to diminish pain and reduce swelling.

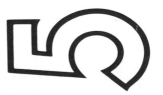

Infections in or around skeletal prosthetic devices. Devices for the total replacement of hips, knees, and finger joints have been used successfully to rehabilitate patients who are severely and painfully disabled. Unfortunately, in some cases these have failed because of infections developing in or around the prosthetic implant.

IN MUSCULOSKELETAL INFECTIONS, PUS OR DRAINAGE FROM THE IN-FECTED SITE IS THE INFECTIVE MATERIAL.

HANDWASHING IS ESSENTIAL:
- *Before and after the care of each patient.*
- *Before and after dressing changes.*
- *Before and after all procedures.*

5

Musculoskeletal System

SITE	ORGANISMS	TYPE STAIN	RELATED DISEASES	SIGNS AND SYMPTOMS
All muscles, bones, and joints	None			
	Any microorganism—bacteria, virus, fungi, parasites—can be pathogenic	As needed for identification	Osteomyelitis	Purulent drainage
				Intermittent pain, locally, with systemic fever
				Edema of local or general area; heat at the site
				Systemic toxicity
				Positive culture with aspiration at site
			Septic (infectious) arthritis	Pus, fever, chills, malaise
				Severe pain in joint
				Tender edema
				Restricted joint movement
				Positive culture with aspiration of joint
			Prosthesis infections	Purulent drainage at site of incision
				Fever
				Persistent pain limiting weight-bearing joint use
				Positive culture with aspiration of site

5

NOTES

SAMPLE AND INSTRUCTIONS FOR CHARTS FOR HOSPITAL, HOME, OFFICE, AND OUTPATIENT CLINIC

Charts for Hospital, Home, Office, and Outpatient Clinic

DISEASE SPECIFIC CODES

ALL At all times
D Desirable, but optional
PH Poor hygiene
SL If soiling likely
SUS If susceptible
WC With contact

DISEASE	CATEGORY SPECIFIC		DISEASE SPECIFIC						
	Type	Duration	Handwashing — Thorough rubbing, lather, rinsing	Private Room Needed	Masks	Gowns	Gloves	Linen — If Soiled, separate	Containers for Body Fluids: Precautions if Contaminated
Common cold									
Adults	-	-	ALL	-	-	-	-	-	-
Infants and children	CI	DI	ALL	ALL	SL	-	-	-	-

HOW TO READ THIS CHART		CATEGORY SPECIFIC CODES	
Steps	**Example**	**Type**	**Duration**
1. Locate infection or disease; read from left to right.	Read first row across as: **Common cold in adults** requires *no special precautions or supplies; handwashing* is required to prevent transmission.	**AFB** Tuberculosis (AFB) isolation	**CN** Off antibiotics; culture negative
2. **Type** indicates *Category Specific* control measures.		**B/BF** Blood/body fluid precautions	**DH** Duration of hospitalization
3. **Duration** signifies length of time to use *Category Specific* control measures.			**DI** Duration of illness/drainage
	Read second row across as: **Common cold in infants and children** can require *contact isolation* for duration of infection; *handwashing* is required to prevent transmission; *private room and gloves* are recommended.	**CI** Contact isolation	**U-a** Until 24 hours after therapy begins
4. Use legend in upper left-hand corner to interpret codes in *Disease Specific* columns.		**D/S** Drainage/secretion precautions	**U-b** Until 2 weeks after therapy begins or until sputa negative
		EP Enteric precautions	**U-c** For 9 days after swelling
		RI Respiratory precautions	**U-d** For 7 days after rash or swelling or onset of infection
5. Column headings in the *Disease Specific* section indicate procedures, patient area, and supplies to be used with *Disease Specific* control measures.		**SI** Strict isolation	**U-e** For 3 days after therapy begins
			U-f For 4 days after rash begins; if immunosuppressed, use DI
			U-g Until HBsAg (hepatitis B surface antigen) is negative
			U-h For 48 hours after effective therapy begins

Charts for Hospital, Home, Office, and Outpatient Clinic

DISEASE SPECIFIC CODES

ALL At all times	**SL** If soiling likely
D Desirable, but optional	**SUS** If susceptible
PH Poor hygiene	**WC** With contact

DISEASE	CATEGORY SPECIFIC		DISEASE SPECIFIC						
	Type	Duration	Handwashing—Thorough rubbing, lather, rinsing	Private Room Needed	Masks	Gowns	Gloves	Linen—if soiled, separate	Containers for body fluids, precautions if Contaminated
Musculoskeletal									
Muscle infections are usually exogenous, produced by trauma (e.g., severe burns, punctures, crushing)	–	–	ALL	✓	✓	✓	✓	✓	✓
Bones—the most common infection is osteomyelitis; exogenous infection may result from surgery (e.g., implants prosthetic devices or trauma)	–	–	ALL	–	–	–	–	–	✓
Deep surgical infection from implants can occur without bone invasion	–	–	ALL	✓	✓	✓	✓	✓	✓

1. Note precautions for specific pathogen (see integumentary system, this reference) usually identified from draining wound in muscular tissue or bony prominence.

Sample Nursing Care Guide

RECOGNITION OF CAUSE OF INFECTION	RESULTS OF CARE PROGRAM	GUIDES FOR ACTION
1. Transmission of infective material: pus or drainage from joint or known prosthesis site.	1. Infective material—pus or drainage from joints or a skeletal prosthesis—will be handled and disposed of properly to prevent transmission.	1. Use thorough handwashing before and after all patient care.
2. Laboratory report of positive culture for infectious process.	2. Auxiliary personnel will be informed of methods of transmission of infection and appropriate cost-effective measures for infection control.	2. Prevent CONTACT with infective material; use gloves and gowns as necessary.
3. Signs and symptoms: ☐ fever ☐ purulent drainage ☐ intermittent pain ☐ chills ☐ joint ache ☐ edema of local or general area	3. Laboratory cultures and antibiotic susceptibility reports reflect efficacy of antibiotic therapy.	3. Dispose of soiled dressings in plastic or heavy paper bag, tie or seal, and place in trash.
4. Knowledge deficit of patient or care givers in any setting for patient care.	4. Current cost-effective measures will be demonstrated daily in patient care practices.	4. Confer with physician and laboratory regarding culture results and antibiotic usage.

Sample Discharge Guide

GENERAL POINTS FOR DISCHARGE	GUIDE FOR CARE IN A CLINIC OR NON-HOSPITAL SETTING	GUIDE FOR CARE IN HOME	GUIDE FOR CARE IN SNF
Information to transmit to anyone receiving a patient with a musculoskeletal infection:	1. Use thorough handwashing before and after all patient care.	1. Use thorough handwashing before and after taking care of patient.	1. Use thorough handwashing before and after all patient care.
1. Identify the source of infection: pus or drainage from a joint or known prosthesis site.	2. Use gloves if there is a possibility of CONTACT with pus or drainage from the infected site.	2. Use gloves if contact with infectious material is possible. Note: Gloves are an expensive item for use in the home by family members. Handwashing if done conscientiously has proved to be sufficient in the home.	2. Use gloves if there is a possibility of CONTACT with pus or drainage.
2. Describe the method of transmission and the infection control measures necessary to prevent CONTACT with infectious material.	3. Use gowns if there is extensive drainage and if soiling of clothing is likely.		3. Use gowns to protect clothing from wound drainage or pus.
	4. Handle dressings carefully. Use NO TOUCH TECHNIQUE when changing dressings on wound or infected site.	3. Wash linens and dishes in usual manner.	4. Handle dressings carefully. Use NO TOUCH TECHNIQUE.
3. Review all medications prescribed.	5. Use plastic or heavy paper bag to dispose of soiled dressings. Tie or seal and place in trash.	4. Use apron or clean towel to cover clothing if drainage is excessive.	5. Place soiled dressings in plastic or heavy paper bag, tie or seal, and dispose of in trash.
4. Notify any agency or transport personnel of special precautions needed to prevent CONTACT with infectious material.	6. Clean surfaces promptly if any soiling occurs. Use approved disinfectant.	5. Handle dressings carefully. Use NO TOUCH TECHNIQUE when changing dressings.	6. Remove tape carefully when removing dressing to prevent skin tearing.
5. Inform public health department if the infection is reportable.		6. Place soiled dressings in plastic or heavy paper bag, tie or seal, and dispose of in trash.	7. Reposition patient carefully to prevent skin burns or shearing.
			8. No special precautions are necessary for linens or dishes.

7. Protect skin from the trauma of tears when tape is removed or when the patient is turned or lifted with sheets.

8. If spills or soiling occurs, clean surfaces with bleach solution diluted 1:10 with water.

9. Clean surfaces promptly if any soiling occurs. Use approved disinfectant.

5

Cost-Effective Measures

The use of proven infection control measures, not rituals, to care for patients with communicable diseases is cost effective. When nursing consistently applies these measures in the health care setting, they reduce infections and death, reduce costs for the facility or patient, reduce potential malpractice suits, facilitate the accreditation process, and strengthen the infection control program as a whole.

When the patient is hospitalized, the following guidelines must be used:

1. Use good handwashing technique at all times.
2. Wash hands before and after taking care of a surgical wound.
3. Do not touch an open or fresh wound directly unless wearing sterile gloves. When wounds are sealed, dressings may be changed without gloves.
4. Drains or closed suction drainage systems should be placed in an adjacent stab wound rather than through the main incisional wound.
5. Dressings over closed wounds should be removed if they are wet or if the patient has signs or symptoms that suggest infection.
6. Culture wound drainage and do a smear for Gram stain.

When the patient is cared for at home, optimum clean techniques are acceptable. The simplest methods to keep the home clean, orderly, and safe are the most practical and cost-effective methods. Rarely will it be necessary to take the ''sterile'' emphasis into the home. The patient will be returning to a known environment where there will be few if any unusual organisms. Handwashing and NO TOUCH TECHNIQUE are the most important factors to emphasize in the home for wound care and drainage secretion and excretion control. These optimum clean techniques will prevent transmission of infective material.

CENTRAL NERVOUS SYSTEM
Guide to Control Infections

The central nervous system (CNS) is that part of the nervous system consisting of the brain, spinal cord, and meninges. Infections in the CNS are devastating and can lead to a variety of debilitating outcomes, including alterations in consciousness and in perceptions of the external environment.

Organisms gain access to the CNS by several routes:

1. Blood circulating from other sites of infection
2. Direct bacterial invasion
3. Devices and/or procedures (e.g., lumbar puncture, intracranial pressure monitoring systems)
4. Surgery or trauma
5. Cerebrospinal fluid shunt systems

The CNS has many anatomical and physiological mechanisms that protect it from infection if they remain intact. Patients with breaks in this system of defense are at the greatest risk.

IN CENTRAL NERVOUS SYSTEM INFECTIONS, BLOOD, SPINAL FLUID, BRAIN TISSUE, AND RESPIRATORY SECRETIONS MAY BE THE INFECTIVE MATERIAL, DEPENDING ON THE ETIOLOGY OF THE DISEASE.

■ *Before and after the care of each patient.*
■ *Before and after the manipulation of shunt junctions or drainage.*
■ *Before and after all procedures*
☐ *After contact with any body secretions or excretions.*

Central Nervous System

SITE	ORGANISMS	TYPE STAIN	RELATED DISEASES	SIGNS AND SYMPTOMS
Brain, spinal cord, and meninges	No normal flora			
	Many microorgan sms—bacteria, viruses, fungi—can be pathogens	As nec. for ID	Meningitis (bacterial or viral), encephalitis	Fever of 10° F or higher and headache, stiff neck
				Alterations in mental function
			Brain abscess	Malaise
				Nausea and vomiting
			Fungal infections	Sinusitis, otitis, and other local URI infections
			Kuru, Creutzfeldt-Jakob disease, and other slow viral infections	Delirium at any stage; may progress to drowsiness, stupor, and coma; coma is associated with a high mortality rate.

SAMPLE AND INSTRUCTIONS FOR
CHARTS FOR HOSPITAL, HOME, OFFICE, AND OUTPATIENT CLINIC

Charts for Hospital, Home, Office, and Outpatient Clinic

DISEASE SPECIFIC CODES

ALL At all times
D Desirable, but optional
PH Poor hygiene

SL If soiling likely
SUS If susceptible
WC With contact

DISEASE	Type	Duration	Handwashing—Thorough Rubbing, Lather, Rinsing	Private Room Needed	Masks	Gowns	Gloves	Linen—if soiled, separate	Containers for Body Fluids; precautions if Contaminated
	CATEGORY SPECIFIC				DISEASE SPECIFIC				
Common cold									
Adults	–	–	ALL	–	–	–	–	–	–
Infants and children	CI	DI	ALL	ALL	SL	–	–	–	–

HOW TO READ THIS CHART		CATEGORY SPECIFIC CODES	
Steps	**Example**	**Type**	**Duration**
1. Locate infection or disease; read from left to right.	Read first row across as: **Common cold in adults** requires *no* special precautions or supplies; handwashing is required to prevent transmission.	**AFB** Tuberculosis (AFB) isolation	**CN** Off antibiotics; culture negative
2. **Type** indicates Category Specific control measures.		**B/BF** Blood/body fluid precautions	**DH** Duration of hospitalization
3. **Duration** signifies length of time to use Category Specific control measures.	Read second row across as: **Common cold in infants and children** can require *contact isolation* for duration of infection; handwashing is required to prevent transmission; *private room and gloves* are recommended.	**CI** Contact isolation	**DI** Duration of illness/drainage
4. Use legend in upper left-hand corner to interpret codes in Disease Specific columns.		**D/S** Drainage/secretion precautions	**U-a** Until 24 hours after therapy begins
5. Column headings in the Disease Specific section indicate procedures, patient area, and supplies to be used with Disease Specific control measures.		**EP** Enteric precautions	**U-b** Until 2 weeks after therapy begins or until sputa negative
		RI Respiratory precautions	**U-c** For 9 days after swelling
		SI Strict isolation	**U-d** For 7 days after rash or swelling or onset of infection
			U-e For 3 days after therapy begins
			U-f For 4 days after rash begins; if immunosuppressed, use DI
			U-g Until HBsAg (hepatitis B surface antigen) is negative
			U-h For 48 hours after effective therapy begins

Charts for Hospital, Home, Office, and Outpatient Clinic

DISEASE SPECIFIC CODES

ALL At all times   SL If soiling likely
D Desirable, but optional   SUS If susceptible
PH Poor hygiene   WC With contact

DISEASE	CATEGORY SPECIFIC		DISEASE SPECIFIC						
	Type	Duration	Handwashing, Thorough rubbing - Lather, rinsing	Private Room Needed	Masks	Gowns	Gloves	Linen - if soiled, separate	Containers for Body fluids: Precautions if Contaminated
Creutzfeldt-Jakob disease[1]	B/BF	DH	ALL	-	-	-	WC	ALL	D
Encephalitis/Encephalomyelitis (suspected; etiology unknown)[2]	EP	U-d	ALL	PH	-	SL	WC	ALL	ALL
Meningitis									
Aseptic[3]	EP	U-d	ALL	PH	-	SL	WC	ALL	ALL
Haemophilus influenzae	RI	U-q	ALL	ALL	-	-	-	-	-
Neisseria meningitidis[3]	RI	U-q	ALL	ALL	-	-	-	-	-

1. Use caution when handling blood, brain tissue, or spinal fluid.
2. Feces are infective.
3. See CDC Guideline for Infection Control for Hospital Personnel or institutional policy regarding employee exposure.

Sample Nursing Care Guide

RECOGNITION OF CAUSE OF INFECTION	RESULTS OF CARE PROGRAM	GUIDES FOR ACTION
1. Transmission of infective material, blood, spinal fluid, brain tissue, respiratory secretions, or feces.	1. Infective material—blood, spinal fluid, brain tissue, respiratory secretions, or feces—will be handled and disposed of properly to prevent transmission.	1. Use thorough handwashing at all times.
2. Laboratory report of positive culture related to disease process.	2. Auxiliary personnel will be informed of methods of transmission of infection and the appropriate cost-effective measures for control.	2. Use gloves if CONTACT with infective material—blood, spinal fluid, brain tissue, respiratory secretions, or feces—is possible.
3. Signs and symptoms: ☐ fever, 101° F or higher ☐ headache ☐ stiff neck ☐ nausea and vomiting ☐ mental changes ☐ delirium ☐ coma ☐ otitis media	3. Current cost-effective measures will be demonstrated in daily patient care practices.	3. Monitor vital signs as frequently as necessary.
		4. Correlate clinical signs with laboratory reports.
		5. Dispose of waste according to policy for infectious process.
4. Knowledge deficit of patient, care givers, transport personnel, or pathology or autopsy personnel, regarding infectious material and method of transmission.		6 Clean spills promptly with bleach solution diluted 1:10 with water.

Sample Discharge Guide

GENERAL POINTS FOR DISCHARGE	GUIDE FOR CARE IN A CLINIC OR NON-HOSPITAL SETTING	GUIDE FOR CARE IN HOME	GUIDE FOR CARE IN SNF
Information to transmit to anyone receiving a patient with a central nervous system infection:	1. Use thorough handwashing before and after all patient care.	1. Use thorough handwashing before and after taking care of patient.	1. Use thorough handwashing before and after all patient care.
1. Identify the source of infection: blood, spinal fluid, brain tissue, feces, respiratory secretions.	2. Use gloves if there is a possibility of CONTACT with infective material.	2. Use gloves if contact with infective material is possible. Note: Gloves are an expensive item for use in the home by family members. Handwashing, if done conscientiously, has proven to be sufficient in the home.	2. Use gloves if there is a possibility of CONTACT with infective material.
2. Describe method of transmission and the infection control measures necessary to prevent contact with infective material.	3. Use gown if soiling is likely.		3. Use gown if soiling is likely.
	4. Use regular toilet to dispose of liquid or solid body waste.	3. Wash linens and dishes in usual manner.	4. No special precautions are necessary for linens or dishes.
3. Review all medication prescribed.	5. Clean surfaces promptly if spills or soiling occur. Use bleach solution diluted 1:10 with water.	4. Use apron or clean towel to cover clothing if patient has drainage.	5. Place soiled dressings or tissues in plastic or heavy paper bag. Tie or seal and place in trash.
4. Notify any agency or transport personnel of special procedures necessary to prevent CONTACT with infective material.	6. Use plastic or heavy paper bag to dispose of soiled dressings or tissues. Tie or seal and place in trash.	5. Handle dressings carefully. Use NO TOUCH TECHNIQUE when changing dressings.	6. Use regular toilet for liquid or solid body waste.
	7. Handle dressing carefully. Use NO TOUCH TECHNIQUE when changing dressings.	6. Place soiled dressings in plastic or heavy paper bag, tie or seal, and dispose of in trash.	7. Use bleach solution diluted 1:10 with water to clean up spills or soiled areas.
5. Inform public health department if infection is reportable.		7. Dispose of liquid or solid body waste in regular toilet.	
		8. Use bleach solution diluted 1:10 with water to clean spills if they occur.	

9

NOTES

Cost-Effective Measures

The use of proven infection control measures, not rituals, to care for patients with communicable diseases is cost effective. When nursing consistently applies these measures in the health care setting, they reduce infections and death, reduce costs for the facility and patient, reduce potential malpractice suits, facilitate the accreditation process, and strengthen the infection control program as a whole.

When the patient is hospitalized, the following guidelines must be used:

1. Use good handwashing technique at all times.
2. When performing invasive procedures, observe sterile technique. VPs and VAs are always placed under operating room conditions. All shunts must be sterile.
3. Keep all invasive systems CLOSED to prevent contamination.
4. Equipment used in the urinary tract or cardiovascular system must be sterile. All catheters should be removed as quickly as possible.
5. Equipment used in the respiratory tract must be sterile, and aspiration must be prevented.
6. Clean all contaminated wounds thoroughly, if possible.

When the patient is cared for at home, optimum clean techniques are acceptable. The simplest methods to keep the home clean, orderly, and safe are the most practical and cost-effective methods. Rarely will it be necessary to take the "sterile" emphasis into the home. The patient will be returning to a known environment where there will be few if any unusual organisms. Handwashing and NO TOUCH TECHNIQUE are the most important factors to emphasize in the home for wound care and drainage secretion and excretion control. These optimum clean techniques will prevent transmission of infectious material.

6

RESPIRATORY SYSTEM
Guide to Control Infections

There are two divisions in the respiratory system. The upper respiratory system includes the air passages above the trachea and is heavily colonized with normal flora. The lower respiratory system includes the bronchial tree and lungs. This area is relatively free of microorganisms.

Introduction of organisms into the lower respiratory system can occur naturally by aspiration or mechanically by devices and procedures used in the treatment of airway blockage or impairment by disease.

IN THE RESPIRATORY SYSTEM, RESPIRATORY SECRETIONS ARE THE INFEC-TIVE MATERIAL.

HANDWASHING IS ESSENTIAL:
- *Before and after the care of each patient.*
- *Before and after any form of tracheostomy care.*
- *Before and after respirator tube drainage.*

7

Respiratory System

SITE	ORGANISMS	TYPE STAIN	RELATED DISEASES	SIGNS AND SYMPTOMS
Upper respiratory system—nose, mouth, throat				*Generally:* Fever, malaise, coryza, rough throat, pharyngitis, otitis media
	Borrelia sp	GN	Relapsing fever	As above
	Fusobacterium sp	GN	Vincent's angina	As above
	Staphylococcus epidermidis	GP	Abscess, otitis media	As above
	Streptococcus salivarius	GP	Mastoiditis, endocarditis	As above
	S. pneumoniae	GP	Pneumonitis, conjunctivitis. meningitis, otitis	As above
	Veillonella sp	GN		—
	Actinomyces israelii	GP	"Lumpy jaw"	Fatal in infants
			Pneumonitis	Lungs involved
	Candida albicans	Yeast	Thrush	"Cotton" mouth
	Corynebacterium sp.	GP		
	Bacteroides sp. (*B. fragilis, B. melaninogenicus, B. oralis*)	GN	Tooth abscess, bacteremia	Sepsis
Lower respiratory system—bronchial tree, lung	No normal flora; many organisms—bacteria, fungi, viruses, parasites—can be pathogenic	As necessary for ID.	Pneumonias, parasitic infections, tuberculosis, fungal infections	Purulent sputa or tracheal drainage Positive x-ray Fever, chills Shortness of breath, cough Positive cultures

SAMPLE AND INSTRUCTIONS FOR CHARTS FOR HOSPITAL, HOME, OFFICE, AND OUTPATIENT CLINIC

Charts for Hospital, Home, Office, and Outpatient Clinic

DISEASE SPECIFIC CODES

ALL	At all times	SL	If soiling likely
D	Desirable, but optional	SUS	If susceptible
PH	Poor hygiene	WC	With contact

DISEASE	CATEGORY SPECIFIC		Handwashing—Thorough rubbing, Lather, Rinsing	Private Room Needed	DISEASE SPECIFIC				
	Type	Duration			Masks	Gowns	Gloves	Linen—if Soiled, separate	Containers for Body Fluids: precautions if Contaminated
Common cold									
Adults	-	-	ALL	-	-	-	-	-	-
Infants and children	CI	DI	ALL	ALL	SL	-	-	-	-

HOW TO READ THIS CHART			CATEGORY SPECIFIC CODES	
Steps	**Example**		**Type**	**Duration**
1. Locate infection or disease; read from left to right.	Read first row across as: **Common cold in adults** *requires no special precautions or supplies; handwashing is required to prevent transmission.*		**AFB** Tuberculosis (AFB) isolation	**CN** Off antibiotics; culture negative
2. **Type** indicates *Category Specific* control measures.			**B/BF** Blood/body fluid precautions	**DH** Duration of hospitalization
3. **Duration** signifies length of time to use *Category Specific* control measures.	Read second row across as: **Common cold in infants and children** can require *contact isolation* for duration of infection; *handwashing* is required to prevent transmission; *private room and gloves* are recommended.		**CI** Contact isolation	**DI** Duration of illness/drainage
			D/S Drainage/ secretion precautions	**U-a** Until 24 hours after therapy begins
4. Use legend in upper left-hand corner to interpret codes in *Disease Specific* columns.				**U-b** Until 2 weeks after therapy begins or until sputa negative
			EP Enteric precautions	**U-c** For 9 days after swelling
5. Column headings in the *Disease Specific* section indicate procedures, patient area, and supplies to be used with *Disease Specific* control measures.			**RI** Respiratory precautions	**U-d** For 7 days after rash or swelling or onset of infection
			SI Strict isolation	**U-e** For 3 days after therapy begins
				U-f For 4 days after rash begins; if immunosuppressed, use DI
				U-g Until HBsAg (hepatitis B surface antigen) is negative
				U-h For 48 hours after effective therapy begins

7

Charts for Hospital, Home, Office, and Outpatient Clinic

DISEASE SPECIFIC CODES

ALL At all times	**SL** If soiling likely
D Desirable, but optional	**SUS** If susceptible
PH Poor hygiene	**WC** With contact

DISEASE	CATEGORY SPECIFIC		Handwashing Thorough Rubbing—Lather, Rinsing	Private Room Needed	DISEASE SPECIFIC				
	Type	Duration			Masks	Gowns	Gloves	Linen—if Soiled, separate	Containers for Body Fluids, Precautions if Contaminated
Adenovirus—infants and young children[1]	CI	DH	ALL	ALL	–	SL	–	D	–
Anthrax (inhaled)	D/S	DI	ALL	–	–	SL	WC	D	D
Aspergillosis	–	–	ALL	–	–	–	–	–	–
Bronchiolitis (etiology unknown)									
Adults	–	–	ALL	–	–	–	–	–	–
Children and infants	CI	DI	ALL	ALL	–	SL	–	D	–
Bronchitis (etiology unknown)									
Adults	–	–	ALL	–	–	–	–	–	–
Children and infants	CI	DI	ALL	ALL	–	SL	–	D	–

	SI	U-d	ALL	ALL	SUS	ALL	ALL	ALL	ALL
Chickenpox (varicella)[2]	D/S	DI	ALL	ALL	—	—	WC	—	D
Chlamydia (respiratory)									
Common cold									
Adults	—	—	ALL	—	—	—	—	—	—
Children and infants	CI	DI	ALL	ALL	—	SL	—	D	—
Congenital rubella[3,4]	CI		ALL	ALL	—	SL	WC	D	D
Corona virus									
Adults	—	—	ALL	—	—	—	—	—	—
Children and infants[5]	CI	DI	ALL	ALL	—	SL	—	D	—
Coxsackie disease[6]	EP/S	U-d	ALL	PH	—	SL	WC	D	D
Croup[7]	CI	DI	ALL	ALL	—	SL	—	D	—
Diphtheria (pharyngeal)	SI	CN	ALL	ALL	ALL	SL	WC	D	D

1. Feces may be infective.
2. Susceptibles should stay out of room. Lesion secretions are infective. Neonates born to mothers with active varicella should be placed in SI at birth. See CDC *Guidelines for Infection Control for Hospital Personnel.*
3. During any admission during first year of life unless nasopharyngeal and urine cultures are negative after 3 months of age.
4. Susceptibles should stay out of room. Pregnant employees may need counseling.
5. Respiratory secretions may be infective.
6. Feces and respiratory secretions may be infective.
7. Viruses such as parainfluenza and influenza A have been associated with this syndrome.

continued

Charts for Hospital, Home, Office, and Outpatient Clinic *continued*

DISEASE SPECIFIC CODES

ALL At all times	**SL** If soiling likely
D Desirable, but optional	**SUS** If susceptible
PH Poor hygiene	**WC** With contact

DISEASE	CATEGORY SPECIFIC		Handwashing—Thorough rubbing, Lather, Rinsing	Private Room Needed	DISEASE SPECIFIC				
	Type	Duration			Masks	Gowns	Gloves	Linen—if Soiled, Separate	Containers for Body Fluids; Precautions if Contaminated
Echovirus (in respiratory secretions and feces)	EP	U-d	ALL	PH	-	SL	WC	D	D
Epiglottitis (*Haemophilus influenzae*)	R	U-a	ALL	ALL	WC	-	-	-	-
Erythema infectiosum	R	U-d	ALL	ALL	WC	-	-	-	-
German measles (rubella)[1]	CI	U-d	ALL	ALL	WC	-	-	-	-
Hemorrhagic fevers[2]	SI	DI	ALL	ALL	ALL	ALL	ALL	ALL	ALL
Herpes Zoster (varicella)—localized; disseminated; or in immunocompromised host[3]	SI	DI	ALL	ALL	SUS	ALL	ALL	ALL	ALL
Influenza and parainfluenza				-					
Adults	-	-	ALL	-	-	-	D	-	-

Children and infants	CI	DI	ALL	ALL	-	SL	-	D	-
Lassa fever	SI	DI	ALL	ALL	ALL	ALL	ALL	ALL	ALL
Marburg virus[2]	SI	DI	ALL	ALL	ALL	ALL	ALL	ALL	ALL
Measles (rubeola)[4]—all types	R	U-f	ALL	ALL	WC	-	-	-	-
Meningitis (respiratory risks)									
Haemophilus influenzae	R	U-a	ALL	ALL	WC	-	-	-	-
Neisseria meningitidis (meningococcal)	R	U-a	ALL	ALL	WC	-	-	-	-
Meningococcal	R	U-a	ALL	ALL	WC	-	-	-	-
Meningococcemia (sepsis)	R	U-a	ALL	ALL	WC	-	-	-	-
Multiply resistant organisms (respiratory)[5]	CI	CN	ALL	ALL	WC	SL	WC	ALL	ALL
Mumps (infectious parotitis)	R	U-c	ALL	ALL	WC	-	-	-	-
Pertussis (whooping cough)	R	U-d	ALL	ALL	WC	-	-	-	-
Parainfluenza virus (infants and young children)	-	-	ALL	ALL	-	SL	-	ALL	-
Pharyngitis (etiology unknown)			ALL						
Adults	-	-	ALL	-	-	-	-	-	-

1. See congenital rubella. Pregnant personnel may need employee counseling. Urine may be infective.
2. Blood/body fluids are infective.
3. Respiratory secretions may be infective.
4. If patient is immunocompromised, maintain "R" for duration of illness.
5. Feces may be infective.

continued

7

Charts for Hospital, Home, Office, and Outpatient Clinic *continued*

DISEASE SPECIFIC CODES

ALL At all times
D Desirable, but optional
PH Poor hygiene

SL If soiling likely
SUS If susceptible
WC With contact

DISEASE	CATEGORY SPECIFIC		DISEASE SPECIFIC						
	Type	Duration	Handwashing—Thorough rubbing, lather, rinsing	Private room Needed	Masks	Gowns	Gloves	Linen—if soiled, separate	Containers for body fluids, precautions if Contaminated
Pharyngitis (etiology unknown) *continued*									
Children and infants	CI	DI	ALL	PH	–	SL	–	D	–
Streptococcus–group A	D/S	U-a	ALL	PH	–	–	–	–	–
Plague, pneumonic	SI	U-e	ALL	ALL	ALL	SL	WC	ALL	ALL
Pneumonia (gram-negative)									
Chlamydia	D/S	DI	ALL	–	–	–	WC	–	D
Etiology unknown[1]	–	–	ALL	–	–	–	–	–	–
Haemophilus influenzae	–	–	ALL	–	–	–	–	–	–
Adults	–	–	ALL	–	–	–	–	–	–

Children and infants	R	U-a	ALL	ALL	WC	-	-	-	-
Legionella	-	-	ALL	-	-	-	-	-	-
Meningococcal	R	U-a	ALL	-	WC	-	-	-	-
Multiply resistant bacterial[2,3,4]	CI	CN	ALL	ALL	WC	SL	WC	ALL	ALL
Staphylococcus aureus[4]	CI	U-a	ALL	ALL	WC	SL	WC	D	D
Streptococcus—group A[4]	CI	U-a	ALL	ALL	WC	SL	WC	D	D
Viral[4]									
Adults	-	-	ALL	-	-	-	-	-	-
Children and infants	CI	DI	ALL	ALL	WC	SL	-	D	-
Rabies	CI	DI	ALL	ALL	WC	SL	WC	D	D
Respiratory syncytial virus (RSV) (Children and infants)	CI	DI	ALL	-	WC	SL	WC	D	D
Rhinovirus (common cold)									
Adults	-	-	ALL	-	-	-	-	-	-
Children and infants	CI	DI	ALL	ALL	-	SL	-	D	-

1. Maintain precautions for most likely etiology.
2. Feces may be infective.
3. See specific agent.
4. Cohorting of infected and colonized patients is acceptable if private rooms are not available.

continued

7

Charts for Hospital, Home, Office, and Outpatient Clinic *continued*

DISEASE SPECIFIC CODES

ALL At all times
D   Desirable, but optional
PH   Poor hygiene

SL   If soiling likely
SUS If susceptible
WC   With contact

DISEASE	CATEGORY SPECIFIC		Handwashing – Thorough rubbing, Lather, Rinsing	Private Room Needed	DISEASE SPECIFIC				
	Type	Duration			Masks	Gowns	Gloves	Linen – if Soiled, separate	Containers for Body Fluids; Precautions if Contaminated
Rubella (German measles)[1,2]	CI	U-d	ALL	ALL	WC	–	–	–	–
Smallpox (variola)[3]	SI	DI	ALL	ALL	WC	ALL	ALL	ALL	ALL
Scarlet fever	D/S	U-a	ALL	PH	–	–	–	–	–
Tuberculosis[4]	AFB	U-b	ALL	ALL	WC/SUS	–	–	–	–
Varicella (chickenpox)[5,6]	SI	U-b	ALL	ALL	WC	ALL	ALL	ALL	ALL
Variola (smallpox)[3]	SI	DI	ALL	ALL	ALL	ALL	ALL	ALL	ALL
Viral diseases									
Pericarditis, myocarditis, or meningitis[7]	EP	U-d	ALL	PH	–	SL	WC	D	D

Respiratory (if not covered elsewhere)								
Adults	-	-	ALL	-	-	-	-	-
Infants and young children	CI	DI	ALL	ALL	-	SL	-	D
Whooping cough (pertussis)	R	U-d	ALL	WC	-	-	-	-

1. Susceptibles should stay out of room. Pregnant employees may need counseling.
2. See congenital rubella. Pregnant personnel may need employee counseling. Urine may be infective.
3. Lesion & respiratory secretions are infective.
4. Confirmed, suspected, laryngeal: sputa is positive or x-ray is suggestive or shows cavity lesion.
5. Feces may be infective.
6. Susceptibles should stay out of room. Lesion secretions are infective. Neonates born to mothers with active varicella should be placed in SI at birth. See *CDC Guidelines for Infection Control for Hospital Personnel.*
7. Feces and possibly respiratory secretions are infectious.

Sample Nursing Care Guide

RECOGNITION OF CAUSE OF INFECTION	RESULTS OF CARE PROGRAM	GUIDES FOR ACTION
1. Transmission of infective material: respiratory secretions, sputum, or pleural drainage. NOTE: Drainage from respirator tubing condensation is infective in patient with a diagnosed infection.	1. Infective respiratory secretions, sputa, or drainage will be handled and disposed of properly to prevent transmission.	1. Thorough handwashing will be done before and after all patient care.
	2. Patient, care givers, or any auxiliary personnel will demonstrate appropriate control measures for respiratory secretions, sputa, or drainage in daily patient care.	2. Gloves will be worn if CONTACT with respiratory secretions is possible.
2. Laboratory report of positive culture for disease process.		3. Mask will be used if infection is identified as aerosoled with suction.
3. Signs and symptoms: *Upper respiratory infection* ☐ fever ☐ rough throat ☐ general malaise ☐ otitis media *Lower respiratory infection* ☐ fever ☐ purulent sputum ☐ chills ☐ cough ☐ shortness of breath ☐ purulent tracheal drainage	3. Infective material will be handled and disposed of properly to prevent transmission. 4. Current cost-effective measures will be demonstrated daily in patient care practices.	4. Suction containers, if not the disposable type, will be kept closed. Empty secretions into regular toilet. 5. Use disposable suction containers when possible. Place in plastic bag. Tie or seal and place in trash. 6. Place dressings or tissues in a plastic or heavy paper bag. Tie or seal and place in trash.
4. Positive chest x-ray.		7. Drain respirator secretions into a *disposable glove.* Place in trash.
5. Knowledge deficit of patient or care givers in any setting, regarding the methods of infection control.		

Sample Discharge Guide

GENERAL POINTS FOR DISCHARGE	GUIDE FOR CARE IN A CLINIC OR NON-HOSPITAL SETTING	GUIDE FOR CARE IN HOME	GUIDE FOR CARE IN SNF
Information to transmit to anyone receiving a patient with a respiratory infection:	1. Use thorough handwashing before and after all patient care.	1. Use thorough handwashing before and after taking care of patient.	1. Use thorough handwashing before and after all patient care.
1. Identify the source of infection: respiratory secretions, sputum or pleural drainage.	2. Use gloves if there is a possibility of CONTACT with respiratory secretions, sputum, or drainage.	2. Place tissues soiled with respiratory secretions or sputum in plastic or heavy paper bag. Tie or seal and place in trash.	2. Use gloves if there is a possibility of CONTACT with respiratory secretions, sputum, or drainage.
2. Describe the method of transmission and ways to prevent contact with infective material.	3. Use masks when working close to patient if required to control disease transmission.	3. Suction procedures may require a disposable catheter. Use for 24 hours, then dispose of in plastic or heavy paper bag. Tie or seal and place in trash.	3. Use masks when working close to patient, if required to control disease transmission.
3. Describe all medications prescribed.	4. Place soiled dressings or tissues in plastic or heavy paper bag. Tie or seal and place in trash.	4. Dispose of dressings in plastic or heavy paper bag. Tie or seal and place in regular trash.	4. Place soiled tissues in plastic or heavy paper bag; seal or tie; place in trash.
4. Notify any agency or transport personnel of special precautions needed to prevent contact with infective material.	5. Flush liquid or solid body wastes down regular toilet.	5. Handle dressings carefully. Use NO TOUCH TECHNIQUE when changing dressings.	5. Clean surfaces promptly if any soiling occurs. Use approved disinfectant.
5. Inform public health department if infection is reportable.	6. Clean surfaces promptly if any soiling occurs. Use an approved disinfectant.	6. Liquids from suction canisters may be flushed down toilet.	6. Use regular toilet for disposal of liquid or solid waste.
		7. If spills or soiling occurs, clean surfaces with bleach solution diluted 1:10 with water.	7. No special precautions necessary for linens or dishes.
			8. Place closed suction drainage container and gloves containing tube condensations into plastic or heavy paper bag. Tie or seal and place in trash.

7

Cost-Effective Measures

The use of proven infection control measures, not rituals, to care for patients with communicable diseases is cost effective. When nursing consistently applies these measures in the health care setting, they reduce infections and death, reduce costs for the facility or patient, reduce potential malpractice suits, facilitate the accreditation process, and strengthen the infection control program as a whole.

When the patient is hospitalized, the following guidelines must be used:

1. Use good handwashing technique at all times.
2. Wash hands before and after contact with patient who is intubated or has had a recent tracheostomy, or after contact with respiratory secretions, whether or not gloves are used.
3. Use only sterile medications.
4. Use only sterile fluids for nebulizers or humidifiers. Discard unused fluids within 24 hours.
5. NEVER add to fluid levels. Always empty and refill. Do not refill reservoirs in advance of use.
6. Patient breathing circuits should be sterile, adequately disinfected, or disposable.
7. Use high-efficiency bacterial filters between collection bottle and vacuum source with portable suction devices (not necessary with wall suction units).
8. Replace patient breathing circuits every 24 hours. Remove fluid buildup carefully to prevent fluid from going into patient's lungs.
9. Change breathing circuits of respiratory equipment between patients.

Tracheostomy Patients

1. Use NO TOUCH TECHNIQUE or sterile gloves when caring for tracheostomy site.
2. Use aseptic technique when changing tube.

Suctioning

1. Suctioning should be done *only* when needed to reduce excessive secretions.
2. Use NO TOUCH TECHNIQUE or gloves on both hands.
3. Use a sterile catheter for *each* series of suctioning.
4. Use only sterile fluid to flush catheter when necessary.
5. Change suction collection tubing between patients.

   When the patient is cared for at home, optimum clean techniques are acceptable. The simplest methods to keep the home clean, orderly, and safe are the most practical and cost-effective methods. Rarely will it be necessary to take the "sterile" emphasis into the home. The patient will be returning to a known environment where there will be few if any unusual organisms. Handwashing and NO TOUCH TECHNIQUE are the most important factors to emphasize in the home for wound care and drainage secretion and excretion control. These optimum clean techniques will prevent transmission of infective material.

IMMUNOSUPPRESSED HOST INFECTIONS
Guide to Control Infections

The compromised/immunosuppressed host is a patient whose normal defense mechanisms are altered by a treatment regimen or a disease process that prevents the normal protective reaction to attack or invasion by bacteria, fungi, or viruses. Body defenses fall into two categories: (1) The nonspecific, which includes the skin, mucous membranes, gastrointestinal tract, respiratory tract, and associated inflammatory responses; and (2) the specific, which includes humoral and cell-mediated immunity, or B- and T-cell immune mechanisms.

Host defenses can be altered in the following ways:

1. *Congenital defects* such as an antibody, cellular, phagocytic, or complement immunodeficiency, or a combination of any or all of these.
2. *Acquired defects* because of extensive burns, bone marrow failure, malfunctioning spleen, allografts, or blood transfusions.
3. *Underlying disease* such as malignant disorders.
4. *Therapeutic treatment modalities* such as chemotherapy and radiation therapy.

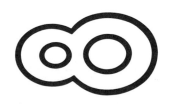

WITH THE IMMUNOSUPPRESSED HOST, THE INFECTIVE MATERIAL IS RE-LATED TO THE ETIOLOGY OF THE DISEASE.

HANDWASHING IS ESSENTIAL:
- *Before and after the care of each patient.*
- *Before and after any treatment or procedure.*

Immunosuppressed Host

SITE	ORGANISMS	TYPE STAIN	RELATED DISEASES	SIGNS AND SYMPTOMS
Any body system is vulnerable	Any microorganism—bacteria, fungi, viruses, yeasts or parasites—can become the pathogen Normal flora is most common agent of infection	As necessary for ID	Various presentations	Note: PUS, the cardinal sign, may not be present. Observe carefully for: Fever—as small as 1° or 2° changes Change in disposition Change in eating habits Change in mental state Hyperventilation Hypotension Systemic dissemination is rapid with viral infections

8

SAMPLE AND INSTRUCTIONS FOR
CHARTS FOR HOSPITAL, HOME, OFFICE, AND OUTPATIENT CLINIC

Charts for Hospital, Home, Office, and Outpatient Clinic

DISEASE SPECIFIC CODES

ALL	At all times	**SL**	If soiling likely
D	Desirable, but optional	**SUS**	If susceptible
PH	Poor hygiene	**WC**	With contact

DISEASE	CATEGORY SPECIFIC		Handwashing—Thorough Rubbing, Lather, Rinsing	Private Room Needed	Masks	Gowns	Gloves	Linen—if Soiled, separate	Containers for Body fluids; Precautions if Contaminated
	Type	Duration					DISEASE SPECIFIC		
Common cold									
Adults	-	-	ALL	-	-	-	-	-	-
Infants and children	CI	DI	ALL	ALL	-	SL	-	-	-

HOW TO READ THIS CHART			CATEGORY SPECIFIC CODES	
Steps	**Example**		**Type**	**Duration**
1. Locate infection or disease; read from left to right.	Read first row across as: **Common cold in adults** *requires no special precautions or supplies; handwashing* is required to prevent transmission.	**AFB** Tuberculosis (AFB) isolation	**CN** Off antibiotics; culture negative
2. **Type** indicates *Category Specific* control measures.		**B/BF** Blood/body fluid precautions	**DH** Duration of hospitalization
3. **Duration** signifies length of time to use *Category Specific* control measures.			**DI** Duration of illness/drainage
			U-a Until 24 hours after therapy begins
	Read second row across as: **Common cold in infants and children** require *contact isolation* for duration of infection; *handwashing* is required to prevent transmission.	**CI** Contact isolation	**U-b** Until 2 weeks after therapy begins or until sputa negative
4. Use legend in upper left-hand corner to interpret codes in *Disease Specific* columns.		**D/S** Drainage/ secretion precautions	**U-c** For 9 days after swelling
			U-d For 7 days after rash or swelling or onset of infection
5. Column headings in the *Disease Specific* section indicate procedures, patient area, and supplies to be used with *Disease Specific* control measures.	*private room and gloves* are recommended.	**EP** Enteric precautions	**U-e** For 3 days after therapy begins
		RI Respiratory precautions	**U-f** For 4 days after rash begins; if immunosuppressed, use DI
		SI Strict isolation	**U-g** Until HBsAg (hepatitis B surface antigen) is negative
			U-h For 48 hours after effective therapy begins

8

111

Charts for Hospital, Home, Office, and Outpatient Clinic

DISEASE SPECIFIC CODES

ALL	At all times	**SL**	If soiling likely
D	Desirable, but optional	**SUS**	If susceptible
PH	Poor hygiene	**WC**	With contact

DISEASE	CATEGORY SPECIFIC		DISEASE SPECIFIC						
	Type	Duration	Handwashing, Thorough Rubbing—Lather; rinsing	Private Room Needed	Masks	Gowns	Gloves	Linen—if Soiled, separate	Containers for Body Fluids; Precautions if Contaminated
Bacterial infections (respiratory, skin, wound)[1]	None	–	ALL	–	–	–	WC	–	–
Viral infections (respiratory, skin, blood)[1]	None	–	ALL	–	–	–	WC	–	–
Systemic infections (disseminated)[1]									
Human immune virus (HIV) (AIDS)	None	–	ALL	PH	–	–	WC	–	–
Cytomegalovirus (CMV)	None	–	ALL	–	–	–	WC	–	–
Herpes simplex, H. zoster[1]	None	–	ALL	–	–	–	WC	–	–
Protozoa									
Pneumocystis carinii (respiratory)[1]	None	–	ALL	–	–	–	WC	–	–
Neutropenia[1]	None	–	ALL	–	–	–	WC	–	–

Strongyloidiasis[2]						WC	
Infants and young children	None	–	ALL	–	–	–	–

1. Reverse isolation has been discontinued. See *Cost-Effective Measures for Immunosuppressed Host*, this section.
2. Respiratory secretions may be infective in immunocompromised host.

8

Sample Nursing Care Guide

RECOGNITION OF CAUSE OF INFECTION	RESULTS OF CARE PROGRAM	GUIDES FOR ACTION
1. Owing to systemic immune deficit this patient is subject to infection from NORMAL FLORA and to possible infection from exogenous (outside) sources.	1. Thorough handwashing will be done before any patient care.	1. Thorough handwashing before any patient care procedure or contact.
2. Laboratory report showing decreased WBCs or agranulocytosis.	2. Patient will practice hand washing regularly.	2. No physical contact with personnel or friends who have known infections. Note: CONTACT is responsible for 95% of infections transmission.
3. Signs and symptoms: ☐ fever ☐ change in mental status ☐ change in eating habits ☐ change in disposition ☐ hypotension ☐ hyperventilation	3. Contact with infections in family and community will be limited.	3. Diet control to limit fresh fruits and vegetables in meals. Wash fruits and vegetables in bleach solution, diluted 1:10 with water. Rinse thoroughly with water.
4. Knowledge deficit of patient and care givers concerning risks for immunosuppressed patients.	4. Current cost-effective measures will be demonstrated daily in patient care practices.	4. Animal contact may need to be limited for immunosuppressed patients due to fecal contamination and to fungal spores on fur.
5. REVERSE ISOLATION is not cost effective and does not prevent contact with normal flora.		

Sample Discharge Guide

GENERAL POINTS FOR DISCHARGE	GUIDE FOR CARE IN A CLINIC OR NON-HOSPITAL SETTING	GUIDE FOR CARE IN HOME	GUIDE FOR CARE IN SNF
Information to transmit to anyone receiving a patient with an immunosuppressed response to infection:	1. Use thorough handwashing before and after all patient care.	1. Use thorough handwashing before and after taking care of patient.	1. Thorough handwashing before and after all patient care.
1. Identify reason for immune deficit: disease process and/or infection.	2. If infection present, use gloves if there is a possibility of CONTACT with infective material.	2. No special precautions are necessary for linens or dishes.	2. No special precautions are necessary for linens or dishes.
2. Describe precautions necessary to protect patient from contact with exogenous sources of infection.	3. Use regular toilet for disposal of liquid or solid body waste.	3. If infection present, place soiled dressings or tissues in plastic or heavy paper bag. Tie or seal and place in trash.	3. If infection is present, use gloves and gowns if there is a possibility of CONTACT with infectious material.
3. Review all medications prescribed.	4. Place soiled dressings in plastic or heavy paper bag. Tie or seal and place in trash.	4. Use regular toilet for disposal of liquid or solid body waste.	4. Place soiled dressings in plastic or heavy paper bag. Tie or seal and place in trash.
4. Notify any agency or transport personnel of special precautions needed to prevent contact with infective material, and vice versa.	5. Counsel patient on need to regulate intake of fresh fruits and vegetables to prevent intestinal colonization with potentially harmful microbes.	5. Regulate amount of fresh vegetables or fruits in patient diet. Wash fruit and vegetables in bleach solution diluted 1:10 with water. Rinse thoroughly with water.	5. Use regular toilet for disposal of liquid or solid waste.
5. Inform public health department if the infection is reportable.	6. Counsel regarding life-style traits that may interfere with control of infection transmission.	6. If infection present, clean surfaces with bleach solution diluted 1:10 with water.	6. If indicated to control disease transmission, clean surfaces promptly with approved disinfectant.
	7. Use gowns if soiling is likely with infective drainage, blood or body fluids.		
	8. If indicated to control disease transmission, clean surfaces with approved disinfectant.		

8

115

Cost-Effective Measures

The use of proven infection control measures, not rituals, to care for patients with communicable diseases is cost effective. When nursing consistently applies these measures in the health care setting, they reduce infections and death, reduce costs for the facility and patient, reduce potential malpractice suits, facilitate the accreditation process, and strengthen the infection control program as a whole.

When the patient is hospitalized, the following guidelines must be used:

1. Limit hospital admissions. Outpatient treatment is encouraged if at all possible.
2. Adequate oral hygiene and skin care must be provided.
3. Environmental factors to be considered:
   ☐ Assigning private rooms
   ☐ Stressing good handwashing technique
   ☐ Providing patient with individual equipment and supplies: NO SHARING WITH OTHER PATIENTS
   ☐ Discouraging eating of fresh fruits and vegetables and contact with fresh flowers or live plants
4. Clinical factors for patient care when hospitalized or at home:
   ☐ Discourage invasive procedures such as urinary and IV catheterization, endotracheal intubation, respiratory assist devices, endoscopy, and bronchoscopy.
   ☐ Devise alternative methods of treatment if at all possible.
5. Sterile technique must be used for ANY invasive procedure.

6. Avoid microabrasions of the skin and surfaces of the mucous membranes from rings, long fingernails, treatments (e.g., rectal temp./suppositories), or sheet burns if patient is assisted in repositioning.

When the patient is cared for at home, optimum clean techniques are acceptable. The simplest methods to keep the home clean, orderly, and safe are the most practical and cost-effective methods. Family members with upper respiratory infections should not care for patient. Wash hands with soap under running water before touching patient. All items in close contact with patient should be clean (e.g., clothes, linens). Soiled disposable items can be disposed of in the regular trash in plastic or heavy paper bags that are sealed or tied shut. Home care techniques must be as clean as possible.

MISCELLANEOUS INFECTIONS
Guide to Control Infections

Miscellaneous infections are a collection of generally rare or unusual infections. The source, cause, and extent of these can be described as miscellaneous.

There is no specific group at risk. Persons over 60 years of age, newborns, infants, young children, and immunocompromised hosts are more susceptible than others. When fever, rash, diarrhea, and persistent URI occur, any of the miscellaneous infections can be suspect and must be correlated with patient history and clinical picture.

IN MISCELLANEOUS INFECTIONS THE INFECTIOUS MATERIAL IS DEPENDENT ON THE ETIOLOGY.

HANDWASHING IS ESSENTIAL:
- *Before and after the care of each patient.*
- *Before and after any procedure with a possibility of contact with infective material.*

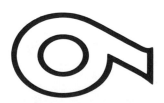

Presentation of Miscellaneous Infections

SITE	ORGANISMS	TYPE STAIN	RELATED DISEASES	SIGNS AND SYMPTOMS
All body systems vulnerable	Any pathogen: bacteria, viruses, fungi, parasites, mold, toxins, zoonosis	As necessary for ID	Various presentations	Spiking fevers
				Rashes, ulcers, lymph abscesses, pustules
				Malaise, chills, headache, cough
				Gastric upset, diarrhea, nausea, vomiting
				Drowsiness, coma, confusion
				Abortion

SAMPLE AND INSTRUCTIONS FOR
CHARTS FOR HOSPITAL, HOME, OFFICE, AND OUTPATIENT CLINIC

Charts for Hospital, Home, Office, and Outpatient Clinic

DISEASE SPECIFIC CODES

ALL	At all times	**SL**	If soiling likely
D	Desirable, but optional	**SUS**	If susceptible
PH	Poor hygiene	**WC**	With contact

DISEASE	CATEGORY SPECIFIC		DISEASE SPECIFIC							
	Type	Duration	Handwashing, Thorough Rubbing—Lather, Rinsing	Private Room Needed	Masks	Gowns	Gloves	Linen—if Soiled, separate	Containers for Body Fluids: Precautions if Contaminated
Common cold										
Adults	–	–	ALL	–	–	–	–	–	–
Infants and children	CI	DI	ALL	ALL	–	SL	–	–	–

HOW TO READ THIS CHART		CATEGORY SPECIFIC CODES	
Steps	**Example**	**Type**	**Duration**
1. Locate infection or disease; read from left to right.	Read first row across as: **Common cold in adults** requires *no* special precautions or supplies; *handwashing* is required to prevent transmission.	**AFB** Tuberculosis (AFB) isolation	**CN** Off antibiotics; culture negative
2. **Type** indicates *Category Specific* control measures.		**B/BF** Blood/body fluid precautions	**DH** Duration of hospitalization
3. **Duration** signifies length of time to use *Category Specific* control measures.	Read second row across as: **Common cold in infants and children** can require *contact isolation* for duration of infection; *handwashing* is required to prevent transmission; *private room and gloves* are recommended.	**CI** Contact isolation	**DI** Duration of illness/drainage
		D/S Drainage/ secretion precautions	**U-a** Until 24 hours after therapy begins
4. Use legend in upper left-hand corner to interpret codes in *Disease Specific* columns.			**U-b** Until 2 weeks after therapy begins or until sputa negative
		EP Enteric precautions	**U-c** For 9 days after swelling
		RI Respiratory precautions	**U-d** For 7 days after rash or swelling or onset of infection
5. Column headings in the *Disease Specific* section indicate procedures, patient area, and supplies to be used with *Disease Specific* control measures.		**SI** Strict isolation	**U-e** For 3 days after therapy begins
			U-f For 4 days after rash begins; if immunosuppressed, use DI
			U-g Until HBsAg (hepatitis B surface antigen) is negative
			U-h For 48 hours after effective therapy begins

121

Charts for Hospital, Home, Office, and Outpatient Clinic

DISEASE SPECIFIC CODES

ALL	At all times	**SL**	If soiling likely
D	Desirable, but optional	**SUS**	If susceptible
PH	Poor hygiene	**WC**	With contact

DISEASE	CATEGORY SPECIFIC		DISEASE SPECIFIC						
	Type	Duration	Handwashing, Thorough Rubbing, Lather, Rinsing	Private Room Needed	Masks	Gowns	Gloves	Linen—if Soiled, separate	Containers for Body Fluids; Precautions if Contaminated
Actinomycosis (all lesions)	–	–	ALL	–	–	–	–	–	–
Amebiasis, liver abscess	–	–	ALL	–	–	–	–	–	–
Arthropod-borne viral fevers (encephalitides—equine eastern, western, Venezuelan equine; encephalomyelitis—St. Louis, Californian)	–	–	ALL	–	–	–	–	–	–
Ascariasis	–	–	ALL	–	–	–	–	–	–
Aspergillosis	–	–	ALL	–	–	–	–	–	–
Blastomycosis (North American—cutaneous or pulmonary)	–	–	ALL	–	–	–	–	–	–
Botulism	–	–		–	–	–	–	–	–
Infant	–	–	ALL	–	–	–	–	–	–

Other						
Candidiasis (all forms; includes mucocutaneous, e.g., moniliasis, thrush)	–	ALL	–	–	–	–
Cat-scratch fever (benign, inoculation, lymphoreticulosis)	–	ALL	–	–	–	–
Chancroid (soft chancre)	–	ALL	–	–	–	–
Clostridium perfringens (food poisoning)	–	ALL	–	–	–	–
Coccidioidomycosis (valley fever)						
Draining lesions[1]	–	ALL	–	WC	–	–
Pneumonia	–	ALL	–	–	–	–
Cryptococcosis	–	ALL	–	–	–	–
Cysticercosis	–	ALL	–	–	–	–
Cytomegalovirus infection (neonatal, immunosuppressed)[2]	–	ALL	–	WC	–	–
Echinococcus (hydatidosis)	–	ALL	–	–	–	–
Epstein-Barr virus infection (any; includes mononucleosis)[3]	–	ALL	–	WC	–	–
Erysipeloid	–	ALL	–	–	–	–

1. Drainage may be infective if spores form.
2. Urine and respiratory secretions may be infective.
3. Respiratory secretions may be infective.

continued

Charts for Hospital, Home, Office, and Outpatient Clinic *continued*

DISEASE SPECIFIC CODES

ALL	At all times	SL If soiling likely
D	Desirable, but optional	SUS If susceptible
PH	Poor hygiene	WC With contact

DISEASE	CATEGORY SPECIFIC		DISEASE SPECIFIC						
	Type	duration	Handwashing—Thorough rubbing, Lather, rinsing	Private Room Needed	Masks	Gowns	Gloves	Linen—if soiled, separate	Containers for body fluids: precautions if Contaminated
Fever of unknown origin (FUO)[1]	-	-	ALL	-	-	-	-	-	-
Food poisoning (see *Clostridium perfringens*)	-	-	ALL	-	-	-	-	-	-
Gonorrhea[2]	-	-	ALL	-	-	-	WC	-	-
Granulocytopenia	-	-	ALL	-	-	-	-	-	-
Granuloma inguinale (donovaniasis, granuloma venereum)[2]	-	-	ALL	-	-	-	WC	-	-
Herpes simplex encephalitis	-	-	ALL	-	-	-	-	-	-
Histoplasmosis (any site)	-	-	ALL	-	-	-	-	-	-
Hookworm disease (ancylostomiasis, uncinariasis)	-	-	ALL	-	-	-	-	-	-
Infectious mononucleosis[3]	-	-	ALL	-	-	-	WC	-	-

Legionnaire's disease[3]	-	ALL	-	-	-	-	-	-
Leprosy	-	ALL	-	-	-	-	-	-
Listeriosis	-	ALL	-	-	-	-	-	-
Lyme disease	-	ALL	-	-	-	-	-	-
Lymphocytic choriomeningitis	-	ALL	-	-	-	-	-	-
Lymphogranuloma venereum	-	ALL	-	-	-	-	-	-
Melioidosis (all forms)[3,2]	-	ALL	-	-	-	-	-	-
Meningitis (bacterial gram-negative)								
Enteric, in neonates[4]	-	ALL	-	-	-	WC	-	-
Fungal	-	ALL	-	-	-	-	-	-
Pneumococcal	-	ALL	-	-	-	-	-	-
Tuberculosis[5]	-	ALL	-	-	-	-	-	-
Other diagnosed bacterial	-	ALL	-	-	-	-	-	-
Molluscum contagiosum	-	ALL	-	-	-	-	-	-
Mucormycosis	-	ALL	-	-	-	-	-	-

1. If signs and symptoms are compatible with (and patient is likely to have) a disease that requires control measures, then use those measures.
2. Drainage/discharge may be infective.
3. Respiratory secretions may be infective.
4. Feces may be infective.
5. If signs of active pulmonary TB, AFB precautions may be necessary. See *Respiratory System*.

continued

Charts for Hospital, Home, Office, and Outpatient Clinic *continued*

DISEASE SPECIFIC CODES

ALL At all times
D Desirable, but optional
PH Poor hygiene

SL If soiling likely
SUS If susceptible
WC With contact

DISEASE	Type	Duration	Handwashing—Thorough Rubbing, Lather, Rinsing	Private Room Needed	Masks	Gowns	Gloves	Linen—if Soiled, separate	Containers for Body Fluids, Precautions if Contaminated
	CATEGORY SPECIFIC				DISEASE SPECIFIC				
Mycobacterium (atypical, pulmonary, wound)[1]	–	–	ALL	–	–	–	WC	–	–
Mycoplasma pneumonia[2]	–	–	ALL	–	–	–	–	–	–
Neutropenia	–	–	ALL	–	–	–	–	–	–
Nocardiosis (draining; other)[3]	–	–	ALL	–	–	–	WC	–	–
Orf[3]	–	–	ALL	–	–	–	WC	–	–
Pinworm infection	–	–	ALL	–	–	–	–	–	–
Pneumonia (not listed elsewhere)									
Bacterial (includes gram-negative)[2]	–	–	ALL	–	–	–	–	–	–
Fungal	–	–	ALL	–	–	–	–	–	–

Legionella[2]	-	-	ALL	-	-	-	WC	-
Mycoplasma (atypical or Eaton)[2]	-	-	ALL	-	-	-	WC	-
Pneumococcal[2]	-	-	ALL	-	-	-	WC	-
Pneumocystis carinii	-	-	ALL	-	-	-	WC	-
Psittacosis (ornithosis)[2]	-	-	ALL	-	-	-	WC	-
Fever	-	-	ALL	-	-	-	-	-
Respiratory infectious disease (acute)								
Adults[2]	-	-	ALL	-	-	-	WC	-
Infants and young children[4]	-	-	ALL	-	-	-	WC	-
Reye syndrome	-	-	ALL	-	-	-	-	-
Rheumatic fever	-	-	ALL	-	-	-	-	-
Rickettsial fevers (tickborne) (Rocky Mt. spotted fever, typhus)[5]	-	-	ALL	-	-	-	WC	-
Rickettsialpox (vesicular rickettsiosis)	-	-	ALL	-	-	-	-	-
Ringworm (dermatophytosis, dermatomycosis, tinea)	-	-	ALL	-	-	-	WC	-
Rocky Mt. spotted fever[5]	-	-	ALL	-	-	-	WC	-

1. Wound drainage may be infective.
2. Respiratory secretions may be infective.
3. Drainage may be infective.
4. Maintain control measures for the bacterial or viral infection most likely.
5. Blood may be infective.

continued

Charts for Hospital, Home, Office, and Outpatient Clinic *continued*

DISEASE SPECIFIC CODES

ALL	At all times	**SL**	If soiling likely
D	Desirable, but optional	**SUS**	If susceptible
PH	Poor hygiene	**WC**	With contact

DISEASE	Type	Duration	Handwashing—Thorough Rubbing, Lather, Rinsing	Private Room Needed	Masks	Gowns	Gloves	Linen—if Soiled, separate	Containers for Body Fluids; precautions if Contaminated
	CATEGORY SPECIFIC					DISEASE SPECIFIC			
Roseola infantum (exanthem subitum)	–	–	ALL	–	–	–	–	–	–
Sporotrichosis	–	–	ALL	–	–	–	–	–	–
Streptococcal disease (Group B)—neonatal[1]	–	–	ALL	–	–	–	–	–	–
Streptococcal disease (not Group A or B) not covered elsewhere	–	–	ALL	–	–	–	–	–	–
Strongyloidiasis[1]	–	–	ALL	–	–	SL	WC	–	–
Syphilis—latent, tertiary (seropositive without lesions)	–	–	ALL	–	–	–	WC	–	–
Tapeworm disease	–	–	ALL	–	–	–	–	–	–
Hymenolepis nana, Taenia solium[1]	–	–	ALL	–	–	–	–	–	–
Other	–	–	ALL	–	–	–	–	–	–

Disease							
Tetanus	–	–	ALL	–	–	–	–
Tinea (fungus, ringworm)[2]	–	–	ALL	–	–	WC	–
Toxoplasmosis	–	–	ALL	–	–	–	–
Trench mouth (Vincent's angina)	–	–	ALL	–	–	–	–
Trichinosis	–	–	ALL	–	–	–	–
Trichomoniasis	–	–	ALL	–	–	–	–
Trichuriasis (whipworm disease)	–	–	ALL	–	–	–	–
Tuberculosis—extra pulmonary							
Meningitis	–	–	ALL	–	–	–	–
Skin test negative—no sign of disease	–	–	ALL	–	–	–	–
Tularemia—pulmonary[3]	–	–	ALL	–	–	–	–
Typhus—endemic/epidemic[4]	–	–	ALL	–	WC	–	–
Urinary tract infection (includes pyelonephritis) with or without urinary catheter[5]	–	–	ALL	–	WC	–	–
Vincent's angina (trench mouth)	–	–	ALL	–	–	–	–
Zygomycosis (phycomycosis, mucormycosis)	–	–	ALL	–	–	–	–

1. Cohorting of infected infants is acceptable. Use gowns and gloves if needed.
2. Includes dermatophytosis, dermatomycosis.
3. Respiratory secretions may be infective.
4. Blood may be infective.
5. See section 3, Genitourinary System, for multiply resistant organisms.

129

Sample Nursing Care Guide

RECOGNITION OF CAUSE OF INFECTION	RESULTS OF CARE PROGRAM	GUIDES FOR ACTION
1. Transmission of infective material; can be from any source (e.g., body site or fluid).	1. Thorough handwashing before and after all patient care will be practiced daily.	1. Thorough handwashing at all times.
2. Laboratory report of positive culture related to disease process.	2. Current cost-effective infection control measures will be demonstrated daily in patient care practices.	2. Follow infection control measures for infection identified.
3. Signs and symptoms: ☐ spiking fevers ☐ chills ☐ malaise ☐ nausea and vomiting ☐ diarrhea ☐ headache ☐ rashes ☐ ulcers ☐ pustules ☐ cough ☐ drowsiness ☐ confusion ☐ coma ☐ spontaneous abortion	3. Infective material will be handled and disposed of properly to prevent transmission.	3. If spills occur, wipe up promptly. Use bleach solution diluted 1:10 with water. 4. Dispose of soiled dressings and tissue in plastic or paper bag. Tie or seal and place in trash. 5. Dispose of drainage or body waste in toilet. 6. Use gowns, gloves, and masks as needed. 7. Follow institutional policy for control of infection identified.
4. Knowledge deficit of patient or care givers or auxiliary personnel concerning cost-effective control of the infection.		

Sample Discharge Guide

GENERAL POINTS FOR DISCHARGE	GUIDE FOR CARE IN A CLINIC OR NON-HOSPITAL SETTING	GUIDE FOR CARE IN HOME	GUIDE FOR CARE IN SNF
Information to transmit to anyone receiving a patient with a miscellaneous infection:	1. Use thorough handwashing before and after all patient care	1. Use thorough handwashing before and after taking care of patient.	1. Use thorough handwashing before and after all patient care.
1. Identify the source of infection: wound drainage, respiratory secretions, blood, body fluids, feces.	2. Use gloves and gowns if there is a possibility of CONTACT with infective material or if soiling of clothing is likely.	2. No special precautions are necessary for linens, dishes, clothing.	2. Use gloves and gowns if there is a possibility of CONTACT with infective material or if soiling of clothing is likely.
2. Describe method of transmission and the infection control measures needed to prevent contact with infective material.	3. Use regular toilet for disposal of liquid or solid body wastes.	3. Use regular toilet for disposal of liquid or solid body wastes.	3. Use masks when working close to patient, if required to control disease transmission.
3. Review all medications prescribed.	4. Place soiled dressings, tissues, etc., in plastic or heavy paper bag. Tie or seal and place in trash.	4. Dispose of soiled tissues, dressings, etc., in plastic or heavy paper bag. Tie or seal and place in trash	4. No special precautions are necessary for linens or dishes.
4. Notify any agency or transport personnel of precautions needed to prevent any contact with infective material.	5. If soiling with infective material occurs, clean surfaces with approved disinfectant. If indicated, use bleach solution diluted 1:10 with water.	5. If spills or soiling occurs, clean surfaces with bleach solution diluted 1:10 with water.	5. Place disposable soiled items in plastic or heavy paper bag. Tie or seal and place in trash.
5. Inform public health department if infection is reportable.	6. Use masks when working close to patient, if required to control disease transmission.		6. Use regular toilet for disposal of liquid or solid body wastes.
			7. If soiling with infective material occurs, clean surfaces with approved disinfectant. If indicated, use bleach solution diluted 1:10 with water.

Cost-Effective Measures

The use of proven infection control measures, not rituals, to care for patients with communicable diseases, is cost effective. When nurses consistently apply updated infection control practice in patient care in any setting, the following results occur:

1. Incidence of infection is reduced.
2. Cost of health care for the facility or patient is reduced.
3. Risk of malpractice suits is reduced.
4. The risk of transmission to the community is reduced.

When the patient is hospitalized, the following guidelines must be used:

1. Thorough handwashing using friction with soap under running water.
2. All waste, dressings, paper goods, disposed of in tied plastic bags in the trash, marked as CONTAMINATED.
3. Soiled linen sent to laundry in bags marked CONTAMINATED.
4. Spills, spatters, gross soiling of floors, bed pans, urinals, emesis basins, drainage containers may be cleaned with a bleach solution of (diluted 1:10 with water).
5. Gloves can be worn if soiling is likely in patient care.

When the patient is cared for at home, optimum clean techniques are acceptable. The simplest methods to keep the home clean, orderly, and safe are the most practical and cost-effective methods. Rarely will it be necessary to take the "sterile" emphasis into the home. The patient will be returning to a known environment where there will be few if any unusual organisms. Handwashing and NO TOUCH TECHNIQUE are the most important factors to emphasize in the home for wound care and drainage secretion and excretion control. These optimum clean techniques will prevent transmission of infective material.

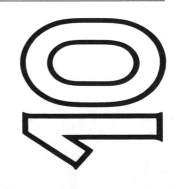

COST-EFFECTIVE MEASURES
FOR INFECTION IN DAY-TO-DAY
PATIENT CARE

Cost-Effective Measures

SPECIAL PRECAUTIONS

ITEM	Hospital/ECF/SNF	Home
Dishes	None	None
Drinking water	None	None
Dressings	All wound dressings should be bagged, labeled and disposed of as infectious waste.	All dressings should be bagged in heavy paper bag, plastic or several thicknesses of newspaper. Dispose of in covered garbage can or trash.
Urine and feces	Flush down toilet	Flush down toilet if municipal or other safe sewage system is used. If flush toilet is NOT available, use health department guidelines.
Needles and syringes	Handle with caution—DO NOT break or recap. DO NOT use needlecutters. Place in prominently labeled, puncture-resistant container and dispose of as infectious waste.	Handle with caution—DO NOT break or recap. DO NOT use needlecutters. Place in prominently labeled, puncture-resistant container (e.g., coffee can or plastic milk carton), place in heavy paper bag and place in covered garbage can, or trash.
Sphygmomanometers and stethoscopes	None	None
Thermometers	Reusable thermometers should be sterilized or receive high level disinfection; otherwise use disposable thermometers.	Do not share with other family members. Store in disinfection solution (70% alcohol) which completely covers the thermometer; or may be stored dry and disinfected for 10 minutes prior to use.

continued

SPECIAL PRECAUTIONS

ITEM	Hospital/ECF/SNF	Home
Linen	Handle gently; place in plastic bag labeled for such linen. Launder according to established procedure.	Wash in family washer. Handle gently; place directly in washer. Use hot water, soap, and 2 cups of bleach. Rinse well to remove all residue. Cover mattresses and pillows with impervious plastic.
Laboratory specimens	Use well-constructed container with a secure lid. Avoid contaminating outside of container. Place in impervious plastic bag for transport.	Same as for hospital ECF/SNF
Patient charts	No contact with infectious material.	
Reusable patient-care equipment	If equipment visibly contaminated, bag label and return for processing.	If equipment visibly contaminated clean with soap and water and bleach solution diluted 1:10 with water.
Disposable patient-care equipment	If visibly contaminated, bag, label, and dispose of as infectious waste.	If visibly contaminated place equipment in plastic bag or several layers of newspaper, or heavy paper bag. Seal and dispose of in trash.
Bagged articles	If articles are visibly contaminated bag in leak proof sturdy color coded bag and return for processing or dispose of as infectious waste.	If articles are visibly contaminated, place disposable items in leak proof plastic bag or several layers of newspapers. Dispose of in trash.
Patient's clothing	Bag and send home or to hospital laundry if soiled with infectious material.	Wash in family washer. Use household bleach. Ironing also reduces pathogens.

Books and magazines	If visibly contaminated, disinfect or dispose of in trash	If visibly contaminated, disinfect with bleach solution diluted 1:10 with water or discard in trash.
Routine cleaning	If surfaces are visibly contaminated, clean with soap and water or approved disinfectant.	If surfaces visibly contaminated, use soap and water with bleach solution diluted 1:10 with water.
Visitors	Two (2) per patient. Instruct in appropriate use of gowns, masks, or other special precautions.	No visitors with infections. Do not overtire patient.
Transportation of infected or colonized patients	Patients should leave room only if necessary. Use appropriate barriers on patient (i.e., masks, gowns, dressings) during treatment.	Instruct family in correct use of barriers (e.g., masks, dressings) on patient being transported.
Terminal cleaning (after infection is cleared)	Clean items in direct contact with patient or in contact with patient's infectious material. Follow established cleaning procedures. *Major cleaning not necessary*	Wipe down *all* horizontal surfaces where soiling may have occurred.
Postmortem handling of bodies	Use same precautions as if patient were still alive; masks are usually not necessary.	Instruct family to call emergency telephone number, follow all instructions. If previous instructions and preparations have been made, follow these.

*Some types of contaminated articles fall into the category of infectious waste and are regulated by state and local guidelines, which apply to hospitals, extended care facilities (ECFs), and skilled nursing facilities (SNFs). Items that become contaminated in home care *do not* fall under special regulations at present. The recommendations in the home care category should be followed to protect members of the family, visitors, public health workers, and visiting nurses.